Hazel O. Torres, CDA, RDA, ~~RW~~ MA
Ann Ehrlich, CDA, MA
Doni Bird, CDA, RDH, MA
Ellen Dietz, CDA, AAS, BS

INSTRUCTOR'S MANUAL TO ACCOMPANY

Modern Dental Assisting

fifth edition

W.B. SAUNDERS COMPANY
A Division of Harcourt Brace & Company
Philadelphia London Toronto Montreal Sydney Tokyo

W.B. Saunders Company
A Division of
Harcourt Brace & Company

The Curtis Center
Independence Square West
Philadelphia, Pennsylvania 19106

Instructor's Manual to accompany
MODERN DENTAL ASSISTING
Fifth Edition

ISBN 0–7216–5054–6

Printed in the United States of America.

Last digit is the print number: 9   8   7   6   5   4   3   2

Instructor's Manual to Accompany
Modern Dental Assisting Text and Workbook, 5th ed
Table of Contents

Learning Objectives

Answer keys

ii

Competency Sheet Evaluation Forms

Introduction to the Instructor's Manual to Accompany Modern Dental Assisting, 5th ed

This manual for use with **Modern Dental Assisting, 5th ed,** and the accompanying workbook contains the following features:

☐ **Learning objectives** for each textbook chapter. These begin on page 1. For student use, these objectives also appear at the beginning of each chapter in the workbook.

☐ **Answer keys** for the exercises in the workbook begin on page 19.

☐ **Evaluation forms** for use with the competency sheets found in the workbook begin on page 28.

Competency Sheets and Evaluation Forms

The use of competency sheets is an important step toward implementing competency-based teaching in a dental assisting curriculum. Through the use of these forms, the student is able to practice and evaluate his or her own performance until mastery (competency) is achieved.

Competency sheets and evaluation forms are also powerful teaching tools. They facilitate giving instant feedback in an objective, measurable manner, and they provide the student with a positive experience in the performance of a technical skill.

Instrumentation lists. Most workbook chapters include one or more competency sheets. When the competency requires instrumentation, a separate page is provided for the student to generate his or her own instrumentation list.

This information can be found in the text or it may be supplied by the instructor. Generating these lists gives the student valuable experience in anticipating **all** of the supplies required for these procedures.

Each sheet provides space for three evaluations. Usually the student does the first as a self-evaluation. Self-evaluation is very important because a qualified dental assistant must be able to judge his or her own skills to know that a technical procedure is being performed correctly and efficiently.

The other spaces are for peer evaluations performed by other students. Serving as evaluators for each other increases learning and student cooperation.

When the student is comfortable with his or her mastery level, it is time to have the instructor and/or clinic supervisor perform a final evaluation. A different evaluation form and format are required for this review.

1. For some competencies, you will want to set a **time limit**. This is based on how quickly an entry-level assistant is expected to perform this procedure.

2. You may want to establish **additional criteria** to determine that the student can competently perform the competency in a clinical setting, within a reasonable time.

3. You'll also need a **scoring system.** Here is an example of how it might work.

   a. Give **2 points** per step.
      These points are awarded *only* if the step is performed correctly.

   b. Based on the number of steps and the points per step, you determine the **total possible score** if all steps are performed correctly.

   c. Then it is necessary to determine the minimum **passing score.**

Of course you'll want to discuss these ground rules and conditions with students before the evaluation process begins.

This manual contains an evaluation form for each clinical competency sheet in the workbook. You will need one copy of this form per student. You are welcome to copy these forms for use in classes where **Modern Dental Assisting, 5th ed,** and the accompanying workbook, are the primary texts.

Learning Objectives for Modern Dental Assisting, 5th ed

Chapter 1 Learning Objectives

- ☐ Trace the development of dentistry in the United States, identify the contributors to this growth, and describe the effect of the Amalgam War on organized dentistry in the United States.

- ☐ Identify the following: G.V. Black, C. Edmund Kells, and Juliette Southard, and describe the contribution of each to the development of dentistry.

- ☐ Discuss the responsibilities, education, and licensure requirements for the general dentist, and describe the eight dental specialties.

- ☐ Describe the primary functions of the dental hygienist, dental assistant, and dental laboratory technician.

- ☐ Discuss the concepts of four-handed and six-handed dentistry.

- ☐ List at least 10 potential extended functions that may be assigned to dental auxiliaries.

- ☐ Identify developments and major contributors to dentistry from early times throughout the world.

Chapter 2 Learning Objectives

- ☐ Describe the responsibilities of the dental assistant, dentist, and other team members to the patients and to each other.

- ☐ State the primary functions of the state dental practice act, the state board of dentistry, and the Dental Assisting National Board.

- ☐ Define the terms: abandonment, acts of commission, acts of omission, duty of care, ethics, jurisprudence, malpractice, negligence, res gestae, and respondeat superior.

- ☐ Differentiate between direct supervision and general supervision.

- ☐ State who may give consent for treatment and discuss ways in which consent may be given.

- ☐ Discuss the ownership of patient records and radiographs within the dental practice.

- ☐ Demonstrate or describe the appropriate way to correct an error in a charting entry.

Chapter 3 Learning Objectives

☐   Describe the body planes, directions, major cavities, and structural units.

☐   Use the appropriate terminology to identify the bones and major landmarks of the skull and face.

☐   Describe the paranasal sinuses and the three divisions of the pharynx.

☐   Identify the structures of the temporomandibular joint and describe its glide and hinge action.

☐   Identify the major muscles of mastication, facial expression, the floor of the mouth, extrinsic muscles of the tongue, and major posterior muscles of the mouth.

☐   Identify the major blood supply and innervation of the face and mouth.

☐   Demonstrate, by pointing or labeling, the major anatomic landmarks of the face and mouth.

Chapter 4 Learning Objectives

☐   Name the three primary embryonic layers and describe the dental tissues each forms following differentiation.

☐   Describe the embryonic development of the palate, including the formation of the primary and secondary palates.

☐   State the effects of genetic and prenatal environmental factors on dental development.

☐   Define modeling, remodeling, deposition, and resorption as they relate to bone and tooth movement.

☐   List the three developmental processes a tooth must go through before it is fully functional.

☐   Describe the tissues of the tooth in terms of structure and function.

☐   List and describe the structures that form the attachment apparatus and the gingival unit.

☐   Describe the characteristics of normal gingival tissue and state the depth of a healthy gingival sulcus.

2

Chapter 5 Learning Objectives

❏ Identify the four types of teeth, describe the specialized functions of each type, classify them as anterior or posterior teeth, and state how many of each are found in the primary and permanent dentition.

❏ Define these terms: curve of Spee and curve of Wilson, the names of the surfaces of the teeth, contours and contacts, overbite and overjet, embrasure, and occlusal form.

❏ Describe Angle's classification of occlusion, including the names of the three classes of occlusion.

❏ Discuss the specialized functions of the primary dentition, state how these teeth differ from those of the permanent dentition, and describe the mixed dentition stage.

❏ Identify the teeth of the primary and permanent dentition using the Universal Numbering System and state the number of cusps and roots of each tooth.

❏ Demonstrate identifying a tooth as to the type, whether it is an anterior or posterior tooth, and whether it is a maxillary or mandibular tooth.

Chapter 6 Learning Objectives

❏ Describe how dental decay occurs and discuss the role of cariogenic foods in dental caries.

❏ Identify the key nutrients, describe their primary functions, define empty calories, and discuss the use of the Food Pyramid as a means of evaluating dietary intake.

❏ List the four key components in preventive dentistry and discuss the roles of systemic and topical fluorides in preventive dentistry.

❏ Describe cheilitis, demineralization, glossitis, remineralization, and scurvy.

❏ Describe the components of plaque, its formation, and patterns of accumulation on the teeth.

❏ Demonstrate personal oral hygiene, including use of a disclosing agent, brushing, flossing, and repeated disclosing.

❏ Demonstrate providing personal oral hygiene instruction to a patient.

Chapter 7 Learning Objectives

❑ Differentiate between psychotic, neurotic, and normal behavior.

❑ Discuss understanding patient behavior in terms of: factors affecting behavior, fear, emotional elements, phobias, and patient responses.

❑ Identify the following coping mechanisms: affiliation, control of the situation, deployment, procrastination, rationalization, rehearsal, and repression.

❑ Differentiate between verbal and nonverbal communication and describe how we communicate nonverbally.

❑ Describe the difference between closed-ended and open-ended questions.

❑ List at least four causes of stress that may occur in the dental office and describe at least four recommended forms of stress reduction.

Chapter 8 Learning Objectives

❑ Describe the child's development through infancy, early childhood, preschool age, and grade school age, as well as differentiate between chronological, mental, and emotional age.

❑ Describe management techniques and precautions when treating the pregnant patient.

❑ Identify at least three special dental problems faced by the older patient.

❑ Describe the role of the dental team in detecting and reporting suspected cases of child, spouse, or geriatric abuse.

❑ Discuss the three major areas in which the assistant aids in providing dental care for a handicapped patient.

❑ Explain the four degrees of intellectual impairment associated with mental retardation.

❑ List at least three problems afflicting infants born with a cleft palate.

❑ Describe the special needs of dental patients with Alzheimer's disease, arthritis, asthma, cardiovascular disorders, diabetes, Down syndrome, epilepsy, muscular dystrophy, and severe kidney disease.

Chapter 9 Learning Objectives

- ❏ Describe the types of medical emergencies that may be encountered in a dental office and discuss the role of staff members in managing these emergencies.

- ❏ Identify the supplies found in a dental office emergency kit and state the purpose of each item.

- ❏ Describe the basic emergency management of anaphylactic reactions, cardiac distress, choking, diabetic emergencies, hemorrhage, seizures, shock, and stroke.

- ❏ Demonstrate taking and recording vital signs.

- ❏ Demonstrate treatment for syncope and postural hypotension.

Chapter 10 Learning Objectives

- ❏ Define the major terms related to microbiology.

- ❏ Describe the roles of host resistance, virulence, and concentration.

- ❏ Name and describe at least five types of disease-producing microorganisms.

- ❏ Discuss at least five modes of disease transmission in the dental office.

- ❏ Describe the actions of the immune system in defending the body.

- ❏ List at least five diseases that are of major concern to dental healthcare workers and state how each is transmitted.

- ❏ Name and describe the four factors that must be present for disease transmission to occur.

Chapter 11 Learning Objectives

☐ Describe four types of oral lesions based on their location in relation to the surface of the tissue.

☐ Name and discuss disturbances in the development of the jaws and in dental development.

☐ Name and discuss diseases of the teeth, periodontal disease, and other diseases of the oral soft tissues.

☐ Describe the symptoms, causes, and treatment of temporomandibular disorders.

☐ Describe three types of oral cancers, state the warning signs and preventive measures, and the dental implications of chemotherapy and radiation treatment.

☐ List and describe at least eight opportunistic infections associated with acquired immunodeficiency syndrome (AIDS) that have oral manifestations.

Chapter 12 Learning Objectives

☐ Describe the role of each of the following federal agencies in relation to the dental healthcare workers and to the dental practice: the Occupational Health and Safety Administration (OSHA), the Centers for Disease Control and Prevention (CDC), and the Environmental Protection Agency (EPA).

☐ List the primary components of a hazard communication program, including the *Bloodborne Pathogens Standard*, and describe their importance to the dental assistant.

☐ Identify the purpose of Material Safety Data Sheets (MSDSs) and hazardous labeling requirements.

☐ Discuss the employer's responsibility in providing hepatitis B vaccination.

☐ Describe the OSHA occupational exposure categories in terms of which workers are included in each category and precautions required for these workers.

☐ In terms of medical waste, differentiate between regulated waste and infectious waste and discuss how each is discarded.

☐ Describe the appropriate handling of hazardous chemicals commonly used in the dental office.

☐ Demonstrate or describe the procedure for cleaning up a spill of potentially infectious material.

Chapter 13 Learning Objectives

❐   Identify the employee exposure risk categories established by the OSHA regulations.

❐   Identify the three classifications of instruments, equipment, and surfaces according to the CDC guidelines.

❐   Define antiseptic, asepsis, bioburden, disinfection, sepsis, and sterilization.

❐   Describe the three major sterilization techniques used in dentistry, as well as the advantages and disadvantages of each.

❐   List and describe the three levels of EPA-approved disinfectants and state when each would be used.

❐   Describe and/or demonstrate the universal precautions and the use of personal protective equipment (PPE).

❐   Demonstrate handwashing before gloving and after removing gloves.

❐   In the sterilization center, locate the contaminated and clean areas and identify the equipment found in each area.

❐   Demonstrate preparing soiled instruments for recirculation. This includes cleaning, wrapping, sterilization, and preset tray preparation.

❐   Demonstrate treatment room cleanup, using the "spray-wipe-spray" method, and treatment room preparation consistent with the CDC guidelines.

Chapter 14 Learning Objectives

❐   Identify and state the use of each major piece of equipment in the dental treatment room.

❐   Describe or demonstrate the care and maintenance of each piece of dental equipment in the treatment room and laboratory.

❐   Demonstrate positioning the operator and assistant for rear, side, and front delivery of care.

❐   Identify and state the use of each major piece of equipment in the dental laboratory.

❐   Describe or demonstrate the morning and evening treatment room routine for the assistant.

❐   Demonstrate admitting, seating, and dismissal of the patient.

Chapter 15 Learning Objectives

❏   Identify the three parts of a dental hand instrument.

❏   Name five types of hand cutting instruments and identify one example of each.

❏   Identify the accessories used in dentistry, including burnishers, spatulas, and scissors.

❏   State the primary use of mandrels, stones, polishing discs, and rubber points.

❏   Describe the use of preset trays and tubs in organizing dental instruments and materials by procedure.

❏   Discuss the special infection control concerns regarding sonic and ultrasonic handpieces.

❏   Demonstrate identifying dental hand instruments.

❏   Demonstrate identifying carbide burs by shape and number series.

❏   Demonstrate identifying types of dental handpieces and state the primary use of each type.

Chapter 16 Learning Objectives

❏   Describe the clock concept of operating zones, explain the uses of each zone, and state where these zones are located when working with a left-handed operator.

❏   Describe the clock concept of operating zones, explain the uses of each zone, and state where these zones are located when working with a right-handed operator.

❏   Discuss hazards and safety precautions involved when transferring instruments.

❏   Demonstrate positioning of the HVE tip.

❏   Demonstrate transferring instruments.

Chapter 17 Learning Objectives

- ☐ Explain the responsibilities of the dentist and assistant relating to dental radiography safety.

- ☐ Describe the properties of x-radiation and explain how cumulative effects damage the body tissues.

- ☐ Identify the radiation exposure control steps taken in the dental practice.

- ☐ Describe the components of a dental x-ray machine and tube head.

- ☐ State how film quality is influenced by time, milliamperage, and kilovoltage.

- ☐ Identify normal anatomic landmarks processing and exposure errors as viewed on radiographs.

- ☐ Demonstrate treatment room preparations before seating the patient for exposing radiographs.

- ☐ Demonstrate producing diagnostic quality radiographs using the paralleling technique and the appropriate film holding devices.

- ☐ Demonstrate processing, mounting, and evaluating radiographs.

Chapter 18 Learning Objectives

- ☐ List and describe the three major steps in diagnosis and treatment.

- ☐ Discuss the assistant's role in diagnosis and treatment planning.

- ☐ List the eight areas of information covered during data gathering and describe the purpose of each.

- ☐ Describe the six clinical observations that are made regarding the patient's appearance.

- ☐ Identify types of cavities based on the cavity classifications as developed by G.V. Black.

- ☐ Identify the names and abbreviations used to describe the tooth surfaces involved in a cavity preparation or restoration.

- ☐ Demonstrate aiding a patient in completing a medical history form.

- ☐ Demonstrate recording the dentist's findings on a tooth diagram during an oral examination.

- ☐ Demonstrate recording scores on a PSR chart.

- ☐ Demonstrate recording patient treatment.

Chapter 19 Learning Objectives

❏   List at least three uses of diagnostic casts.

❏   Discuss the differences between reversible and irreversible hydrocolloids and describe the two phases of all hydrocolloids.

❏   Explain why alginate impressions are not stored in water or exposed to the air.

❏   State the recommended water-powder ratios for model plaster, dental stone, and high-strength dental stone.

❏   List at least three factors that influence the setting time of gypsum products.

❏   Describe or demonstrate the procedure for obtaining a wax-bite registration.

❏   Demonstrate obtaining maxillary and mandibular alginate impressions.

❏   Demonstrate pouring, trimming, finishing, polishing, and labeling maxillary and mandibular diagnostic casts.

Chapter 20 Learning Objectives

❏   Identify, by schedule, the major drugs covered by the Controlled Substance Act.

❏   Identify the major routes of drug administration and describe the procedures to be followed when handling medications.

❏   Describe three types of drugs used in dentistry for the control of anxiety, and differentiate between mild, moderate, and strong analgesics, giving an example of each.

❏   Describe the specialized uses and potential side effects (in dentistry) of the antibiotics penicillin, tetracycline, and erythromycin.

❏   Describe the uses of vasoconstrictors, corticosteriods, and atropine sulfate.

❏   Describe obtaining local anesthesia by block and by infiltration injection techniques.

❏   Identify the four stages of general anesthesia and describe the agents most commonly used to produce general anesthesia.

❏   Identify the three planes of nitrous oxide sedation in dentistry and identify the steps to be taken if the patient moves into the wrong plane.

❏   Demonstrate the placement of topical anesthetic ointment prior to an injection of a local anesthetic solution on the maxillary and mandibular arches.

❏   Demonstrate the preparation of an aspirating local anesthetic syringe, the proper disposal of the used needle, and the care of the used syringe.

10

Chapter 21 Learning Objectives

- ❐ Explain the difference between a prophylaxis and coronal polishing.

- ❐ State at least three indications and three contraindications for coronal polish.

- ❐ Name and describe five types of extrinsic stains found on the teeth.

- ❐ Describe the two categories of intrinsic stains found in the teeth.

- ❐ Name the tooth surfaces where a rubber cup is used, and those where a bristle brush is used.

- ❐ Describe the technique for using a prophy angle in terms of the grasp, handpiece speed, and positioning against the tooth.

- ❐ Describe at least four types of abrasives used in polishing teeth and state when each is used.

- ❐ Describe or demonstrate on each quadrant establishing a fulcrum or finger rest during coronal polishing.

- ❐ Describe or demonstrate proper operator and assistant seating for each quadrant during coronal polishing.

- ❐ In states where it is legal, demonstrate, on a typodont, coronal polishing technique.

Chapter 22 Learning Objectives

- ❐ List at least eight indications for use of the dental dam.

- ❐ Identify the instruments used in dental dam preparation, placement, and removal.

- ❐ Describe the placement of a dental dam over a fixed bridge, placement with cervical ligature, use of the QuickDam, and placement with a cervical clamp.

- ❐ Demonstrate punching a dental dam for placement on the maxillary anterior teeth and for mandibular posterior placement.

- ❐ Demonstrate assisting in the placement of a dental dam.

- ❐ Demonstrate assisting in the removal of a dental dam.

Chapter 23 Learning Objectives

❏   List at least five factors that affect dental materials.

❏   Describe the steps in enamel bonding.

❏   Define smear layer and state why it is important in dentin bonding.

❏   List at least four types of dental cements and state the uses of each.

❏   Identify the important characteristics, uses, and means of manipulation of zinc phosphate, zinc oxide-eugenol, IRM, and glass ionomer cements.

❏   Describe the three types of fillers used in composite restorative materials and state when each is preferred. Also explain the differences between light-cured and self-cured composite restorative materials.

❏   Identify the major components of an amalgam alloy.

❏   Discuss the use and placement of cavity liners and bases.

❏   Demonstrate dispensing and mixing of the most commonly used dental cements either for luting a cast restoration or for use as a protective base.

Chapter 24 Learning Objectives

❏   List the uses of custom trays and discuss the materials used to construct them.

❏   Differentiate between light-bodied, medium-bodied, and heavy-bodied elastomeric impression materials and state one use of each.

❏   Explain the purpose of the occlusal registration and describe the use of the triple tray technique to obtain this impression.

❏   Demonstrate the construction and finishing of a custom impression tray.

❏   Demonstrate the preparation of at least two types of elastomeric impression materials.

❏   Demonstrate assisting during the two-step impression technique, using silicone impression materials.

Chapter 25 Learning Objectives

- ❏ Define the terms cavity walls, line angles, point angles, and describe the principles of cavity preparation.

- ❏ State the steps in bonding an amalgam restoration.

- ❏ Describe the placement of direct bonded composite veneers.

- ❏ Discuss the preparation, application, and removal of a matrix for a Class II amalgam restoration and for a Class II composite restoration.

- ❏ Describe the materials and the procedure for in-office and night guard bleaching of vital teeth.

- ❏ Identify the instrumentation required for the placement of a Class III composite restoration and a Class II amalgam restoration.

- ❏ Demonstrate the role of a chairside assistant in the preparation and placement of a Class II amalgam restoration.

- ❏ Demonstrate the role of a chairside assistant in the preparation and placement of a Class III composite restoration.

Chapter 26 Learning Objectives

- ❏ State the roles of the registered dental hygienist and dental assistant in periodontics.

- ❏ Describe the steps in a complete periodontal examination.

- ❏ Identify the specialized instruments used in periodontics.

- ❏ Describe these periodontal procedures: prophylaxis, scaling and curettage, root planing, gingivectomy, gingivoplasty, and osteoplasty.

- ❏ Discuss the points to be covered when giving postoperative instructions to a patient following periodontal surgery.

- ❏ Demonstrate preparing an instrument tray for periodontal surgery.

- ❏ Demonstrate mixing noneugenol periodontal surgical dressing.

Chapter 27 Learning Objectives

❒   Describe the services provided in a pediatric dental practice.

❒   Identify the parts of an examination for a child patient and state why each part is important.

❒   List the classifications used to identify the degree of fracture of an anterior tooth.

❒   Describe the process of fabricating a stainless steel crown and state the assistant's role in this procedure.

❒   Discuss the types of pulpal therapy for both primary and young permanent teeth.

❒   If it is legal in your state, demonstrate the topical application of fluoride gel.

❒   If it is legal in your state, demonstrate the application of pit and fissure sealant on an extracted natural tooth.

Chapter 28 Learning Objectives

❒   Describe the factors affecting malocclusion and the phases of orthodontic treatment.

❒   Identify the specialized instruments used in orthodontic treatment.

❒   Identify the diagnostic records that must be gathered before orthodontic treatment planning, including the use of cephalometric radiographs and measurements.

❒   Describe the types of fixed and removable appliances used in orthodontic treatment.

❒   Describe the types and the selection, adaptation, cementation, and removal of orthodontic bands.

❒   Describe the placement and removal of bonded orthodontic brackets.

❒   Demonstrate the placement and removal of elastomeric ring orthodontic separators.

❒   Demonstrate assisting in the cementation of orthodontic bands with zinc phosphate cement.

Chapter 29 Learning Objectives

- ❏ State the indications and contraindications for endodontic treatment.
- ❏ Identify the specialized instruments used in endodontic treatment.
- ❏ Describe the specialized diagnostic tests used in an endodontic examination.
- ❏ Explain why dental dam is required during endodontic treatment.
- ❏ Discuss the specialized local anesthesia techniques that may be used during endodontic treatment.
- ❏ Describe the steps in endodontic treatment.
- ❏ Demonstrate performing a pulp vitality test on a normal tooth using an electric pulp tester.

Chapter 30 Learning Objectives

- ❏ Explain the difference between a general dentist and an oral and maxillofacial surgeon (OMFS) and list the procedures most commonly performed by an OMFS.
- ❏ Describe the role of the dental assistant in surgical procedures.
- ❏ State the difference between incisional and excisional biopsies.
- ❏ Name the two types of dental implants approved by the American Dental Association (ADA).
- ❏ Discuss the indications and contraindications for dental implants.
- ❏ Describe the home care procedures required for dental implants.
- ❏ Describe the two stages of surgery for placement of osseointegrated dental implants.
- ❏ Demonstrate identifying the specialized instruments used for common surgical procedures.

Chapter 31 Learning Objectives

- ☐ Name indications and contraindications for fixed prosthetics.
- ☐ Differentiate between noble and base metals and discuss their use in dental alloys.
- ☐ Describe the differences between full crowns, inlays, onlays, and veneer crowns.
- ☐ Identify the components of a fixed bridge.
- ☐ Describe the function of temporary coverage for a fixed bridge.
- ☐ Describe the use of retraction cord prior to taking a final impression.
- ☐ Discuss the uses of core build-ups, pins, and posts in crown retention.
- ☐ Demonstrate creating provisional coverage for a tooth with a crown preparation.

Chapter 32 Learning Objectives

- ☐ Differentiate between a complete and partial denture.
- ☐ Describe the indications and contraindications for removable partial and complete dentures.
- ☐ List the components of a partial and complete denture.
- ☐ Describe the steps in the construction of a removable partial denture.
- ☐ Discuss the steps in the construction of a complete denture.
- ☐ Describe the construction of an overdenture and an immediate denture.
- ☐ Describe the process of relining or repairing a complete or partial denture.
- ☐ Demonstrate taking an alginate impression on edentulous mandibular and maxillary arches.

16

Chapter 33 Learning Objectives

❏ Describe how marketing applies to a dental practice and differentiate between internal and external marketing.

❏ Discuss the steps in outlining the appointment book and in making appointment entries.

❏ Describe how to schedule appointments for the following: children, emergency patients, new patients, recall patients, and utilizing an EFDA.

❏ Identify how to use these filing systems: alphabetical, numerical, cross-reference, chronological, and subject.

❏ Name three types of preventive recall systems and state the benefits of each.

❏ Demonstrate professional telephone courtesy.

❏ Demonstrate the proper procedure for greeting patients.

Chapter 34 Learning Objectives

❏ Describe the basic components of both manual and computerized accounts receivable management systems.

❏ Discuss the role of the office manager/business assistant in making financial arrangements and in preventive account management.

❏ List at least three different types of dental insurance plans and describe the factors that limit the patient's benefits under these plans.

❏ Discuss the steps in claims preparation, the use of American Dental Association procedure codes, and the application of the birthday rule when children have dual coverage.

❏ Demonstrate making financial arrangements with a patient.

❏ Demonstrate making a telephone collection call on an overdue account.

Chapter 35 Learning Objectives

☐ Describe the accounts payable management functions in the dental office, including the procedures for handling COD deliveries and petty cash.

☐ Discuss how to manage inventory control, how to establish the reorder point, and reorder quantity for a specified dental supply item.

☐ State the four factors that should be checked prior to making an equipment service repair call.

☐ State the proper way to handle an NSF check and describe the steps required to make the necessary adjustments in the practice and patient account records.

☐ Identify common payroll taxes, describing which are withheld from the employee's pay, which are the financial responsibility of the employer, and which require matching contributions.

☐ Describe the steps in reconciling a bank statement.

Chapter 36 Learning Objectives

☐ Identify at least three sources where a dental assistant may find information about potential employment opportunities.

☐ Describe at least three types of employment opportunities for the dental assistant.

☐ Describe suitable attire for an employment interview.

☐ Identify two important functions when greeting or being dismissed by the interviewer.

☐ Describe the responsibilities of the employee and the employer in maintaining employment in the dental office.

☐ Discuss the elements of an employment agreement.

☐ Demonstrate being interviewed for a position as a chairside assistant.

18

Answer Keys to Accompany
Modern Dental Assisting Workbook, 5th ed

Chapter 1		Chapter 2		Chapter 3		Chapter 4	
1.	D	1.	B	1.	D	1.	D
2.	A	2.	B	2.	A	2.	D
3.	F	3.	D	3.	B	3.	D
4.	B	4.	A	4.	A	4.	C
5.	C	5.	C	5.	D	5.	B
6.	A	6.	D	6.	E	6.	C
7.	D	7.	C	7.	B	7.	A
8.	D	8.	D	8.	A	8.	C
9.	B	9.	B	9.	B	9.	B
10.	C	10.	C	10.	A	10.	D
11.	D	11.	A	11.	C	11.	C
12.	A	12.	D	12.	A	12.	C
13.	D	13.	D	13.	A	13.	B
14.	C	14.	D	14.	B	14.	C
15.	D	15.	B	15.	C	15.	B
16.	D	16.	A	16.	B	16.	C
17.	D	17.	A	17.	D	17.	B
18.	D	18.	A	18.	C	18.	B
19.	D	19.	D	19.	C	19.	B
20.	A	20.	B	20.	B	20.	B
21.	D	21.	C	21.	A	21.	C
22.	A	22.	D	22.	C	22.	B
23.	C	23.	D	23.	A	23.	B
24.	B	24.	A	24.	A	24.	A
25.	B	25.	C	25.	C	25.	D

Chapter 5		Chapter 6		Chapter 7		Chapter 8	
1.	C	1.	D	1.	D	1.	C
2.	A	2.	B	2.	C	2.	B
3.	C	3.	B	3.	A	3.	C
4.	A	4.	A	4.	D	4.	D
5.	A	5.	C	5.	D	5.	C
6.	A	6.	C	6.	B	6.	A
7.	A	7.	B	7.	D	7.	B
8.	C	8.	D	8.	D	8.	B
9.	D	9.	C	9.	A	9.	A
10.	A	10.	B	10.	D	10.	D
11.	D	11.	D	11.	A	11.	B
12.	B	12.	B	12.	D	12.	A
13.	B	13.	B	13.	D	13.	B
14.	C	14.	B	14.	D	14.	C
15.	A	15.	C	15.	D	15.	A
16.	B	16.	B	16.	D	16.	A
17.	D	17.	A	17.	B	17.	B
18.	A	18.	C	18.	A	18.	A
19.	C	19.	A	19.	D	19.	C
20.	A	20.	B	20.	D	20.	C
21.	B	21.	D	21.	C	21.	B
22.	D	22.	C	22.	D	22.	B
23.	A	23.	B	23.	B	23.	D
24.	C	24.	A	24.	D	24.	A
25.	C	25.	B	25.	D	25.	B

Chapter 9		Chapter 10		Chapter 11		Chapter 12	
1.	A	1.	D	1.	A	1.	D
2.	A	2.	A	2.	A	2.	B
3.	D	3.	D	3.	C	3.	B
4.	B	4.	C	4.	C	4.	C
5.	A	5.	D	5.	C	5.	D
6.	A	6.	C	6.	B	6.	C
7.	A	7.	C	7.	B	7.	A
8.	D	8.	C	8.	A	8.	B
9.	B	9.	B	9.	A	9.	C
10.	C	10.	B	10.	B	10.	B
11.	A	11.	A	11.	D	11.	B
12.	B	12.	A	12.	D	12.	D
13.	B	13.	B	13.	A	13.	A
14.	D	14.	D	14.	A	14.	D
15.	B	15.	A	15.	B	15.	C
16.	C	16.	D	16.	C	16.	C
17.	C	17.	D	17.	A	17.	B
18.	A	18.	A	18.	D	18.	D
19.	D	19.	A	19.	B	19.	D
20.	B	20.	B	20.	A	20.	D
21.	C	21.	A	21.	B	21.	A
22.	D	22.	C	22.	A	22.	D
23.	B	23.	D	23.	B	23.	B
24.	C	24.	C	24.	A	24.	C
25.	A	25.	D	25.	D	25.	A

Chapter 13		Chapter 14		Chapter 15		Chapter 16	
1.	C	1.	D	1.	C	1.	C
2.	A	2.	A	2.	D	2.	C
3.	A	3.	B	3.	B	3.	A
4.	B	4.	B	4.	C	4.	A
5.	D	5.	A	5.	D	5.	D
6.	C	6.	A	6.	D	6.	D
7.	A	7.	A	7.	A	7.	B
8.	B	8.	C	8.	D	8.	D
9.	B	9.	B	9.	B	9.	B
10.	A	10.	A	10.	A	10.	A
11.	D	11.	A	11.	D	11.	C
12.	A	12.	C	12.	A	12.	A
13.	A	13.	D	13.	B	13.	C
14.	D	14.	A	14.	B	14.	B
15.	B	15.	D	15.	A	15.	D
16.	C	16.	B	16.	A	16.	B
17.	B	17.	B	17.	B	17.	C
18.	A	18.	B	18.	A	18.	A
19.	D	19.	B	19.	B	19.	A
20.	D	20.	D	20.	C	20.	B
21.	D	21.	D	21.	A	21.	C
22.	A	22.	D	22.	D	22.	A
23.	B	23.	B	23.	C	23.	D
24.	D	24.	A	24.	D	24.	C
25.	B	25.	B	25.	A	25.	D

Chapter 17		Chapter 18		Chapter 19		Chapter 20	
1.	D	1.	D	1.	D	1.	A
2.	D	2.	C	2.	A	2.	B
3.	C	3.	D	3.	D	3.	D
4.	A	4.	D	4.	C	4.	B
5.	D	5.	A	5.	B	5.	B
6.	C	6.	D	6.	B	6.	C
7.	C	7.	A	7.	C	7.	B
8.	D	8.	C	8.	B	8.	A
9.	B	9.	D	9.	B	9.	D
10.	D	10.	E	10.	B	10.	D
11.	D	11.	B	11.	A	11.	B
12.	A	12.	C	12.	B	12.	B
13.	B	13.	F	13.	D	13.	A
14.	A	14.	B	14.	A	14.	A
15.	D	15.	B	15.	B	15.	D
16.	C	16.	C	16.	B	16.	B
17.	B	17.	A	17.	B	17.	D
18.	B	18.	D	18.	B	18.	B
19.	B	19.	C	19.	A	19.	C
20.	B	20.	B	20.	C	20.	B
21.	D	21.	D	21.	B	21.	D
22.	B	22.	A	22.	B	22.	D
23.	A	23.	C	23.	A	23.	A
24.	C	24.	B	24.	D	24.	B
25.	A	25.	D	25.	D	25.	D

Chapter 21		Chapter 22		Chapter 23		Chapter 24	
1.	D	1.	D	1.	D	1.	C
2.	A	2.	B	2.	B	2.	B
3.	B	3.	A	3.	B	3.	C
4.	D	4.	D	4.	C	4.	B
5.	A	5.	D	5.	D	5.	D
6.	C	6.	C	6.	B	6.	A
7.	B	7.	B	7.	D	7.	A
8.	B	8.	D	8.	B	8.	A
9.	C	9.	D	9.	D	9.	C
10.	B	10.	C	10.	B	10.	B
11.	D	11.	B	11.	B	11.	B
12.	D	12.	C	12.	C	12.	D
13.	D	13.	A	13.	C	13.	B
14.	A	14.	A	14.	B	14.	C
15.	D	15.	D	15.	A	15.	D
16.	A	16.	D	16.	B	16.	A
17.	D	17.	C	17.	B	17.	A
18.	B	18.	C	18.	A	18.	B
19.	D	19.	B	19.	D	19.	D
20.	B	20.	C	20.	A	20.	C
21.	A	21.	D	21.	B	21.	B
22.	D	22.	B	22.	B	22.	B
23.	A	23.	D	23.	D	23.	C
24.	D	24.	B	24.	B	24.	C
25.	B	25.	B	25.	D	25.	C

Chapter 25		Chapter 26		Chapter 27		Chapter 28	
1.	A	1.	D	1.	D	1.	D
2.	A	2.	B	2.	A	2.	D
3.	D	3.	D	3.	C	3.	D
4.	B	4.	C	4.	A	4.	A
5.	A	5.	D	5.	B	5.	D
6.	B	6.	D	6.	C	6.	A
7.	A	7.	C	7.	C	7.	B
8.	C	8.	D	8.	A	8.	B
9.	A	9.	D	9.	A	9.	D
10.	C	10.	A	10.	D	10.	B
11.	C	11.	B	11.	B	11.	A
12.	A	12.	C	12.	D	12.	B
13.	B	13.	A	13.	B	13.	C
14.	B	14.	A	14.	B	14.	B
15.	D	15.	C	15.	A	15.	D
16.	A	16.	C	16.	A	16.	B
17.	B	17.	B	17.	C	17.	B
18.	A	18.	B	18.	C	18.	A
19.	D	19.	A	19.	D	19.	D
20.	B	20.	C	20.	B	20.	D
21.	B	21.	A	21.	A	21.	B
22.	C	22.	D	22.	C	22.	D
23.	A	23.	C	23.	A	23.	B
24.	A	24.	A	24.	C	24.	C
25.	A	25.	B	25.	D	25.	B

Chapter 29		Chapter 30		Chapter 31		Chapter 32	
1.	B	1.	D	1.	C	1.	D
2.	C	2.	A	2.	B	2.	B
3.	C	3.	B	3.	B	3.	A
4.	D	4.	C	4.	C	4.	A
5.	D	5.	C	5.	A	5.	D
6.	D	6.	D	6.	C	6.	D
7.	D	7.	B	7.	B	7.	B
8.	D	8.	D	8.	D	8.	B
9.	A	9.	A	9.	A	9.	B
10.	D	10.	C	10.	B	10.	B
11.	D	11.	A	11.	C	11.	A
12.	C	12.	D	12.	D	12.	C
13.	B	13.	A	13.	C	13.	C
14.	C	14.	D	14.	A	14.	D
15.	C	15.	C	15.	D	15.	B
16.	B	16.	A	16.	D	16.	B
17.	A	17.	D	17.	B	17.	D
18.	A	18.	C	18.	D	18.	A
19.	C	19.	A	19.	B	19.	D
20.	B	20.	C	20.	B	20.	C
21.	D	21.	D	21.	D	21.	D
22.	B	22.	B	22.	C	22.	B
23.	B	23.	A	23.	C	23.	B
24.	A	24.	C	24.	A	24.	D
25.	C	25.	D	25.	B	25.	B

Chapter 33		Chapter 34		Chapter 35		Chapter 36	
1.	C	1.	C	1.	B	1.	C
2.	B	2.	B	2.	A	2.	B
3.	C	3.	D	3.	B	3.	D
4.	D	4.	A	4.	D	4.	B
5.	B	5.	A	5.	C	5.	C
6.	C	6.	A	6.	D	6.	D
7.	D	7.	B	7.	A	7.	C
8.	A	8.	C	8.	C	8.	D
9.	D	9.	A	9.	C	9.	A
10.	B	10.	A	10.	D	10.	B
11.	B	11.	B	11.	D	11.	C
12.	B	12.	C	12.	A	12.	C
13.	A	13.	D	13.	C	13.	D
14.	B	14.	A	14.	B	14.	B
15.	B	15.	A	15.	C	15.	C
16.	D	16.	D	16.	B	16.	D
17.	C	17.	C	17.	C	17.	A
18.	B	18.	B	18.	B	18.	B
19.	D	19.	D	19.	C	19.	B
20.	C	20.	B	20.	A	20.	C
21.	D	21.	A	21.	A	21.	D
22.	A	22.	D	22.	B	22.	B
23.	D	23.	D	23.	D	23.	C
24.	B	24.	D	24.	D	24.	A
25.	C	25.	C	25.	A	25.	D

Instrumentation List for _____

Circle the appropriate icons if these
items would be used in actual patient
care.

List below all instruments, materials, and supplies required for this
procedure.

_____   _____

_____   _____

_____   _____

_____   _____

_____   _____

_____   _____

_____   _____

_____   _____

_____   _____

_____   _____

_____   _____

Evaluation Form

Competency 3 - 1 *Identifying Anatomic Landmarks of the Face (1)*

Performance Objective: When working with another student, or through the use of a mannikin or photograph, the student will identify the landmarks of the face as listed below.

Note: If working with a person, the student will point but not touch the face.

Time limit: _____ *Other conditions:* _____

Points per step = _____ *Maximum score =* _____ *Passing score =* _____

---

*Check the left box **only** if step is performed correctly.*
Place score in the adjacent box.

	Evaluator #1	Evaluator #2
1. Identified the ala of the nose.	☐ ☐	☐ ☐
2. Identified the inner canthus of the eye.	☐ ☐	☐ ☐
3. Identified the outer canthus of the eye.	☐ ☐	☐ ☐
4. Identified the commissures of the lips.	☐ ☐	☐ ☐
5. Identified the midline (midsagittal plane).	☐ ☐	☐ ☐

Student's score _____ _____

Evaluator's comments

Evaluation Form

Competency 3 - 2 *Identifying Anatomic Landmarks of the Face (2)*

Performance Objective: When working with another student, or through the use of a mannikin or photograph, the student will identify the landmarks of the face as listed below.

Note: If working with a person, the student will point but not touch the face.

Time limit: _____ Other conditions: _____

Points per step = _____ Maximum score = _____ Passing score = _____

Check the left box **only** if step is performed correctly.
Place score in the adjacent box.

	Evaluator #1	Evaluator #2
1. Identified the nasion.	☐ ☐	☐ ☐
2. Identified the philtrum.	☐ ☐	☐ ☐
3. Identified the tragus of the ear.	☐ ☐	☐ ☐
4. Identified the vermilion border.	☐ ☐	☐ ☐
5. Identified the zygomatic arch	☐ ☐	☐ ☐

Student's score _____ _____

Evaluator's comments

Evaluation Form

Competency 5 - 1 *Identifying Types of Teeth*

Performance Objective: Given five teeth, the student will identify each tooth as to the type, and classify each as to whether it is an anterior or a posterior tooth.

Note: This is an entry-level skill. Students are expected to continue to improve their skills until they can identify any tooth in the permanent or primary dentition and state whether it comes from the maxillary or mandibular arch.

Important: *The instructor will supply the teeth to be identified. These will be from a typodont or sterilized extracted teeth and will be lettered A, B, C, D, and E. No additional instrumentation is required for this procedure.*

Time limit: _____ Other conditions: _____

Points per step = _____ Maximum score = _____ Passing score = _____

Check the left box **only** if step is performed correctly. Place score in the adjacent box.

			Evaluator #1	Evaluator #2
1.	**Tooth A:**	Identified type of tooth.	☐ ☐	☐ ☐
2.	**Tooth A:**	Identified it correctly as an anterior or a posterior tooth.	☐ ☐	☐ ☐
3.	**Tooth B:**	Identified type of tooth.	☐ ☐	☐ ☐
4.	**Tooth B:**	Identified it correctly as an anterior or a posterior tooth.	☐ ☐	☐ ☐
5.	**Tooth C:**	Identified type of tooth.	☐ ☐	☐ ☐
6.	**Tooth C:**	Identified it correctly as an anterior or a posterior tooth.	☐ ☐	☐ ☐
7.	**Tooth D:**	Identified type of tooth.	☐ ☐	☐ ☐
8.	**Tooth D:**	Identified it correctly as an anterior or a posterior tooth.	☐ ☐	☐ ☐
9.	**Tooth E:**	Identified type of tooth.	☐ ☐	☐ ☐
10.	**Tooth E:**	Identified it correctly as an anterior or a posterior tooth.	☐ ☐	☐ ☐

Student's score _____   _____

Evaluator's comments

Evaluation Form

Competency 5 - 2 *Identifying Permanent Teeth*

Performance Objective: The student will identify each tooth as to the type of tooth it is, and state whether it is a maxillary or mandibular tooth.

Important: *The instructor will supply five sterilized extracted teeth, or typodont teeth with roots. These will be labeled A, B, C, D, E. No additional instrumentation is required for this procedure.*

Time limit: _____ Other conditions: _____

Points per step = _____ Maximum score = _____ Passing score = _____

*Check the left box **only** if step is performed correctly.*
Place score in the adjacent box.

	Evaluator #1	Evaluator #2
1. **Tooth A:** Stated the type of tooth.	☐ ☐	☐ ☐
2. **Tooth A:** Identified it as a maxillary or mandibular tooth.	☐ ☐	☐ ☐
3. **Tooth B:** Stated the type of tooth.	☐ ☐	☐ ☐
4. **Tooth B:** Identified it as a maxillary or mandibular tooth.	☐ ☐	☐ ☐
5. **Tooth C:** Stated the type of tooth.	☐ ☐	☐ ☐
6. **Tooth C:** Identified it as a maxillary or mandibular tooth.	☐ ☐	☐ ☐
7. **Tooth D:** Stated the type of tooth.	☐ ☐	☐ ☐
8. **Tooth D:** Identified it as a maxillary or mandibular tooth.	☐ ☐	☐ ☐
9. **Tooth E:** Stated the type of tooth.	☐ ☐	☐ ☐
10. **Tooth E:** Identified it as a maxillary or mandibular tooth.	☐ ☐	☐ ☐

Student's score   _____   _____

Evaluator's comments

Evaluation Form

Competency 6 - 1 *Demonstrating Personal Oral Hygiene*

Performance Objective: The student will demonstrate his or her personal oral hygiene skills by using disclosing solution, then flossing and brushing. Upon completion, disclosing solution is applied again to demonstrate that all plaque has been removed.

Important: *The student will need disclosing solution (or tablets), a toothbrush, toothpaste (optional), dental floss, and other aids as indicated by the instructor.*

Time limit: _____ Other conditions: _____

Points per step = _____ Maximum score = _____ Passing score = _____

Check the left box **only** if step is performed correctly.
Place score in the adjacent box.

	Evaluator #1		Evaluator #2	
1. Used disclosing agent to disclose plaque.	☐	☐	☐	☐
2. Brushed teeth without trauma to the gingiva.	☐	☐	☐	☐
3. Used floss removing remaining plaque without trauma to the gingiva.	☐	☐	☐	☐
4. Used other aids as indicated by the instructor.	☐	☐	☐	☐
5. Repeated use of disclosing agent indicated that all plaque has been removed.	☐	☐	☐	☐

Student's score _____ _____

Evaluator's comments

Evaluation Form

Competency 6 - 2 *Teaching Personal Oral Hygiene Skills*

Performance Objective: The student will demonstrate the use of disclosing solution (or tablets), toothbrushing, and dental floss to remove plaque without injury to the gingiva.

Note: Gloves are not worn during this procedure because the assistant does not place his or her hands in the patient's mouth.

Important: *The student may use a large model and toothbrush for the demonstration. The "patient" should be supplied with disclosing solution or tablets, a new toothbrush, and dental floss.*

Time limit: _____ Other conditions: _____

Points per step = _____ Maximum score = _____ Passing score = _____

*Check the left box **only** if step is performed correctly. Place score in the adjacent box.*

	Evaluator #1	Evaluator #2
1. Gathered appropriate supplies.	☐ ☐	☐ ☐
2. Explained the procedure to the patient.	☐ ☐	☐ ☐
3. Explained the use of the disclosing agent and instructed the patient how to use it.	☐ ☐	☐ ☐
4. Observed patient during use of the disclosing agent and made constructive suggestions as necessary.	☐ ☐	☐ ☐
5. Instructed patient in toothbrushing.	☐ ☐	☐ ☐
6. Observed patient during toothbrushing and made constructive suggestions as necessary.	☐ ☐	☐ ☐
7. Instructed patient in the use of dental floss.	☐ ☐	☐ ☐
8. Observed patient during flossing and made constructive suggestions as necessary.	☐ ☐	☐ ☐
9. Had patient reapply disclosing agent.	☐ ☐	☐ ☐
10. Congratulated and encouraged the patient when efforts were successful.	☐ ☐	☐ ☐

Student's score _____ _____

Evaluator's comments

34

Evaluation Form

Competency 9 - 1 *Providing Emergency Treatment of Syncope*

Performance Objective: The student will demonstrate emergency care for a patient in a state of syncope in the dental chair. The patient is breathing and has no visible sign of injury or distress.

Important: *This will be performed in a treatment room with another student playing the role of the patient. A first aid kit, ammonia ampules, and gauze sponges should be available.*

Time limit: _____ Other conditions: _____

Points per step = _____ Maximum score = _____ Passing score = _____

*Check the left box **only** if step is performed correctly. Place score in the adjacent box.*

	Evaluator #1	Evaluator #2
1. Asked patient, "Are you all right?" The patient did not respond.	☐ ☐	☐ ☐
2. Called for help without alarming other patients.	☐ ☐	☐ ☐
3. Placed patient in supine position with head slightly lower than his feet.	☐ ☐	☐ ☐
4. Placed an ammonia ampule in a gauze sponge, then crushed the ampule.	☐ ☐	☐ ☐
5. Wafted the ampule near, but not directly under, the patient's nose.	☐ ☐	☐ ☐
6. Reassured patient as he regained consciousness.	☐ ☐	☐ ☐

Student's score _____ _____

Evaluator's comments

Evaluation Form

Competency 9 - 2 *Taking and Recording Blood Pressure*

Performance Objective: The student will demonstrate taking and recording a patient's blood pressure.

Important: *A sphygmomanometer and a stethoscope are required for this procedure.*

Time limit: _____ Other conditions: _____

Points per step = _____ Maximum score = _____ Passing score = _____

Check the left box **only** if step is performed correctly.
Place score in the adjacent box.

	Evaluator #1		Evaluator #2	
1. Gathered appropriate supplies.	☐	☐	☐	☐
2. Explained procedure to the patient.	☐	☐	☐	☐
3. Placed blood pressure cuff appropriately on the patient's arm.	☐	☐	☐	☐
4. Placed stethoscope correctly in his or her ears.	☐	☐	☐	☐
5. Placed the diaphragm of the stethoscope just above the elbow on the patient's brachial artery.	☐	☐	☐	☐
6. Inflated the cuff and obtained systolic pressure reading.	☐	☐	☐	☐
7. Deflated the cuff slowly and obtained diastolic pressure reading.	☐	☐	☐	☐
8. Removed cuff and recorded readings.	☐	☐	☐	☐
9. Prepared equipment for return to storage.	☐	☐	☐	☐

Student's score _____ _____

Evaluator's comments

Evaluation Form

Competency 12 - 1 *Cleaning Up a Simulated Infectious Materials Spill*

Performance Objective: The student will use the appropriate exposure control methods to clean up a simulated spill of potentially infectious liquid on a hard surface floor.

Time limit: _____ Other conditions: _____

Points per step = _____ Maximum score = _____ Passing score = _____

Check the left box **only** if step is performed correctly.
Place score in the adjacent box.

	Evaluator #1	Evaluator #2
1. Gathered appropriate supplies.	☐ ☐	☐ ☐
2. Washed hands, put on utility gloves and other appropriate PPE.	☐ ☐	☐ ☐
3. Wet the area with a suitable disinfectant.	☐ ☐	☐ ☐
4. Used a large wad of paper towels to wipe up area.	☐ ☐	☐ ☐
5. Did not allow gloves to touch liquid and discarded towels appropriately after use.	☐ ☐	☐ ☐
6. Applied disinfectant again and stated how long the area should be left wet.	☐ ☐	☐ ☐
7. Dried the area with fresh paper towels and discarded the towels appropriately.	☐ ☐	☐ ☐
8. Removed gloves without touching contaminated outside.	☐ ☐	☐ ☐
9. Washed hands immediately and stated how utility gloves should be prepared for reuse.	☐ ☐	☐ ☐
10. Followed the appropriate exposure control measures throughout the procedure.	☐ ☐	☐ ☐

Student's score _____ _____

Evaluator's comments

37

Evaluation Form

Competency 13 - 1 *Handwashing Before Gloving*

Performance Objective: Given the appropriate setting and equipment, the student will demonstrate handwashing before gloving.

Important: *A sink and handwashing supplies are required for this procedure.*

Time limit: _____ *Other conditions:* _____

Points per step = _____ *Maximum score =* _____ *Passing score =* _____

*Check the left box **only** if step is performed correctly.*
Place score in the adjacent box.

	Evaluator #1	Evaluator #2
1. Gathered appropriate supplies.	☐ ☐	☐ ☐
2. Before gloving, removed all jewelry, including watch and rings.	☐ ☐	☐ ☐
3. Regulated flow so the water was warm.	☐ ☐	☐ ☐
4. Dispensed liquid soap and scrubbed hands vigorously.	☐ ☐	☐ ☐
5. Rinsed, then scrubbed again.	☐ ☐	☐ ☐
6. Worked soap under fingernails. If beginning of day, used orangewood stick and nail brush.	☐ ☐	☐ ☐
7. Rinsed hands with cool water.	☐ ☐	☐ ☐
8. Used a paper towel to dry hands and then forearms.	☐ ☐	☐ ☐
9. If necessary, used towel to turn off water.	☐ ☐	☐ ☐
10. Followed the appropriate exposure control measures throughout the procedure.	☐ ☐	☐ ☐

Student's score   _____   _____

Evaluator's comments

Evaluation Form

Competency 13 - 2 *Cleaning a Treatment Room After Patient Care*

Performance Objective: The student will discard waste appropriately and use the "spray-wipe-spray" method to clean soiled surfaces in a treatment room. (The tray of soiled instruments has already been returned to the sterilization center.)

Time limit: _____ Other conditions: _____

Points per step = _____ Maximum score = _____ Passing score = _____

*Check the left box **only** if step is performed correctly.*
Place score in the adjacent box.

	Evaluator #1		Evaluator #2	
1. Gathered appropriate supplies.	☐	☐	☐	☐
2. Washed hands and put on appropriate PPE.	☐	☐	☐	☐
3. Removed soiled barriers.	☐	☐	☐	☐
4. Sprayed soiled surface with a cleaning solution.	☐	☐	☐	☐
5. Vigorously wiped surface after spraying.	☐	☐	☐	☐
6. Sprayed surface with a disinfecting solution.	☐	☐	☐	☐
7. Repeated steps 4, 5, and 6 until all soiled surfaces had been cleaned and disinfected.	☐	☐	☐	☐
8. Discarded waste appropriately.	☐	☐	☐	☐
9. Removed PPE and washed hands.	☐	☐	☐	☐
10. Followed the appropriate exposure control measures throughout the procedure.	☐	☐	☐	☐

Student's score _____   _____

Evaluator's comments

Evaluation Form

Competency 13 - 3 *Preparing a Treatment Room for Patient Care*

Performance Objective: The student will complete all of the steps required in preparing the treatment room prior to seating the patient.

Time limit: _____ Other conditions: _____

Points per step = _____ Maximum score = _____ Passing score = _____

*Check the left box **only** if step is performed correctly.*
Place score in the adjacent box.

	Evaluator #1	Evaluator #2
1. Gathered appropriate supplies.	☐ ☐	☐ ☐
2. Placed clean barriers.	☐ ☐	☐ ☐
3. Prepared the patient's chart, radiographs, and laboratory work.	☐ ☐	☐ ☐
4. Determined that the treatment room was ready with the dental chair in the proper position.	☐ ☐	☐ ☐
5. Determined that all hoses and cords were out of the patient's way.	☐ ☐	☐ ☐
6. Placed sterile instrument tray for next patient.	☐ ☐	☐ ☐
7. Followed the appropriate exposure control measures throughout the procedure.	☐ ☐	☐ ☐

Student's score _____ _____

Evaluator's comments

Evaluation Form

Competency 13 - 4 *Preparing Instruments for Recirculation*

Performance Objective: Provided with a tray of soiled instruments and the appropriate sterilization center equipment, the student will clean, wrap, sterilize (by autoclaving), and reassemble the contents of the instrument tray.

Time limit: _____	*Other conditions:* _____
Points per step = _____	*Maximum score =* _____ *Passing score =* _____

*Check the left box **only** if step is performed correctly.*
Place score in the adjacent box.

	Evaluator #1	Evaluator #2
1. Gathered appropriate supplies.	☐ ☐	☐ ☐
2. Washed hands and put on appropriate PPE.	☐ ☐	☐ ☐
3. Discarded waste appropriately.	☐ ☐	☐ ☐
4. Placed instruments in carrier, rinsed, and then ran through ultrasonic cycle.	☐ ☐	☐ ☐
5. Rinsed instruments, removed from carrier, and placed on towel to dry.	☐ ☐	☐ ☐
6. Bagged and sealed instruments for autoclaving.	☐ ☐	☐ ☐
7. Either ran autoclave, or simulated same. Stated the time, pressure, and temperature required.	☐ ☐	☐ ☐
8. Disinfected tray, removed PPE, and washed hands.	☐ ☐	☐ ☐
9. Removed cool sterile instruments from autoclave and reassembled tray with all appropriate supplies.	☐ ☐	☐ ☐
10. Followed the appropriate exposure control measures throughout the procedure.	☐ ☐	☐ ☐

Student's score _____   _____

Evaluator's comments

Evaluation Form

Competency 14 - 1 *Identifying Treatment Room Equipment*

Performance Objective: The student will identify and state the purpose of each of the following major pieces of equipment in a dental treatment room: the dental chair, operating light, operator's stool, assistant's stool. The student will also be able to identify the dental unit(s) and carts, and the attachments included on each.

Important: *This procedure is to be performed in a dental treatment room. No additional instrumentation is required.*

Time limit: _____ Other conditions: _____

Points per step = _____ Maximum score = _____ Passing score = _____

*Check the left box **only** if step is performed correctly.*
Place score in the adjacent box.

	Evaluator #1	Evaluator #2
1. Demonstrated adjusting the height of the dental chair and placing it in the upright position.	☐ ☐	☐ ☐
2. Demonstrated adjusting the operating light so it does not shine in the patient's eyes.	☐ ☐	☐ ☐
3. Identified the operator's stool and the assistant's stool.	☐ ☐	☐ ☐
4. Demonstrated the correct seated position of the assistant.	☐ ☐	☐ ☐
5. Identified the assistant's unit or cart and identified the attachments on it.	☐ ☐	☐ ☐
6. Identified the operator's unit or cart and identified the attachments on it.	☐ ☐	☐ ☐
7. Identified the radiographic view box.	☐ ☐	☐ ☐
8. Identified the curing light.	☐ ☐	☐ ☐
9. Identified the amalgamator.	☐ ☐	☐ ☐
10. Identified the sharps container.	☐ ☐	☐ ☐

Student's score   _____   _____

Evaluator's comments

Evaluation Form

Competency 14 - 2 *Seating and Positioning the Patient*

Performance Objective: The student will demonstrate seating the patient, placing the patient napkin, and placing the patient in the supine position.

Important: *A treatment room setting, a patient, a supply of patient towels, and a towel clip are required for this procedure.*

Time limit: _____ Other conditions: _____

Points per step = _____ Maximum score = _____ Passing score = _____

Check the left box **only** if step is performed correctly.
Place score in the adjacent box.

	Evaluator #1	Evaluator #2
1. Determined that the appropriate barriers were in place in the treatment room.	☐ ☐	☐ ☐
2. Determined that the dental chair was in the proper position and other equipment out of the way.	☐ ☐	☐ ☐
3. Determined that the patient chart, radiographs, and laboratory work were in place.	☐ ☐	☐ ☐
4. Determined that the appropriate tray was in place.	☐ ☐	☐ ☐
5. Escorted the patient to the treatment room.	☐ ☐	☐ ☐
6. Seated the patient, placed personal objects (such as a handbag or glasses) in a safe place.	☐ ☐	☐ ☐
7. If patient is female, asked her to remove lipstick.	☐ ☐	☐ ☐
8. Cautioned patient before adjusting the chair position.	☐ ☐	☐ ☐
9. Positioned chair so that the patient was in a supine position.	☐ ☐	☐ ☐
10. Maintained patient comfort throughout.	☐ ☐	☐ ☐

Student's score _____ _____

Evaluator's comments

Evaluation Form

Competency 15 - 1 *Identifying Dental Hand Instruments*

Performance Objective: Given an assortment of dental hand instruments, the student will identify each type of instrument. (The instructor may choose to give bonus points for correct identification of the primary use of each instrument.)

Important: *The instructor will prepare assorted hand instruments to be identified by numbering them from 1 through 10.*

Time limit: _____	Other conditions: _____
Points per step = _____	Maximum score = _____ Passing score = _____

*Check the left box **only** if step is performed correctly.*
Place score in the adjacent box.

	Evaluator #1	Evaluator #2
1. Correctly identified instrument #1.	☐ ☐	☐ ☐
2. Correctly identified instrument #2.	☐ ☐	☐ ☐
3. Correctly identified instrument #3.	☐ ☐	☐ ☐
4. Correctly identified instrument #4.	☐ ☐	☐ ☐
5. Correctly identified instrument #5.	☐ ☐	☐ ☐
6. Correctly identified instrument #6.	☐ ☐	☐ ☐
7. Correctly identified instrument #7.	☐ ☐	☐ ☐
8. Correctly identified instrument #8.	☐ ☐	☐ ☐
9. Correctly identified instrument #9.	☐ ☐	☐ ☐
10. Correctly identified instrument #10.	☐ ☐	☐ ☐

Student's score   _____   _____

Evaluator's comments

Evaluation Form

Competency 15 - 2 *Identifying Dental Handpieces and Burs*

Performance Objective: The student will identify types of handpieces and burs (by shape). (The instructor may choose to give bonus points for correct identification of the number series for each type of bur.)

Important: *The instructor will prepare three handpieces (numbered 1 through 3) and seven basic burs (numbered 4 through 10).*

Time limit: _____ Other conditions: _____

Points per step = _____ Maximum score = _____ Passing score = _____

*Check the left box **only** if step is performed correctly.*
Place score in the adjacent box.

	Evaluator #1	Evaluator #2
1. Identified the type of handpiece #1.	☐ ☐	☐ ☐
2. Identified the type of handpiece #2.	☐ ☐	☐ ☐
3. Identified the type of handpiece #3.	☐ ☐	☐ ☐
4. Identified the shape of bur #4.	☐ ☐	☐ ☐
5. Identified the shape of bur #5.	☐ ☐	☐ ☐
6. Identified the shape of bur #6.	☐ ☐	☐ ☐
7. Identified the shape of bur #7.	☐ ☐	☐ ☐
8. Identified the shape of bur #8.	☐ ☐	☐ ☐
9. Identified the shape of bur #9.	☐ ☐	☐ ☐
10. Identified the shape of bur #10.	☐ ☐	☐ ☐

Student's score _____ _____

Evaluator's comments

Evaluation Form

Competency 16 - 1 *Positioning the HVE Tip*

Performance Objective: In a simulation, the student will demonstrate HVE tip placement for each area of the mouth

Important: *Required for this procedure are: a patient or manikin, a dental chair, a sterile HVE tip, sterile cotton rolls, and a sterile mouth mirror. Appropriate PPE is also required. It is desirable to have someone play the role of the operator.*

Time limit: _____ Other conditions: _____

Points per step = _____ Maximum score = _____ Passing score = _____

*Check the left box **only** if step is performed correctly. Place score in the adjacent box.*

	Evaluator #1	Evaluator #2
1. Gathered appropriate supplies.	☐ ☐	☐ ☐
2. Positioned HVE tip appropriately for maxillary right quadrant.	☐ ☐	☐ ☐
3. Positioned HVE tip appropriately for maxillary left quadrant.	☐ ☐	☐ ☐
4. Positioned HVE tip appropriately for maxillary anterior area.	☐ ☐	☐ ☐
5. Positioned HVE tip appropriately for mandibular right quadrant.	☐ ☐	☐ ☐
6. Positioned HVE tip appropriately for mandibular left quadrant.	☐ ☐	☐ ☐
7. Positioned HVE tip appropriately for mandibular anterior area.	☐ ☐	☐ ☐
8. Followed the appropriate exposure control measures throughout the procedure.	☐ ☐	☐ ☐

Student's score   _____   _____

Evaluator's comments

46

Competency 16 - 2 *Exchanging Dental Instruments*

Performance Objective: The student will demonstrate the exchange of dental instruments in a safe and efficient manner with the working end delivered in the position of use.

Important: *The instruments to be exchanged are determined by the instructor including examples of pen and palm grasp instruments. The instruments should be numbered from 1 through 10.*

Time limit: _____ Other conditions: _____

Points per step = _____ Maximum score = _____ Passing score = _____

Check the left box **only** if step is performed correctly.
Place score in the adjacent box.

	Evaluator #1	Evaluator #2
1. Passed instrument #1 in an acceptable manner.	☐ ☐	☐ ☐
2. Passed instrument #2 in an acceptable manner.	☐ ☐	☐ ☐
3. Passed instrument #3 in an acceptable manner.	☐ ☐	☐ ☐
4. Passed instrument #4 in an acceptable manner.	☐ ☐	☐ ☐
5. Passed instrument #5 in an acceptable manner.	☐ ☐	☐ ☐
6. Passed instrument #6 in an acceptable manner.	☐ ☐	☐ ☐
7. Passed instrument #7 in an acceptable manner.	☐ ☐	☐ ☐
8. Passed instrument #8 in an acceptable manner.	☐ ☐	☐ ☐
9. Passed instrument #9 in an acceptable manner.	☐ ☐	☐ ☐
10. Passed instrument #10 in an acceptable manner.	☐ ☐	☐ ☐
11. Followed the appropriate exposure control measures throughout the procedure.	☐ ☐	☐ ☐

Student's score   _____   _____

Evaluator's comments

Evaluation Form

Competency 17 - 1 *Exposing an Adult Radiographic Survey*
Using the Paralleling Technique

Performance Objective: The student will use the paralleling technique to produce a complete diagnostic quality radiographic survey. The number and types of exposures in the series are to be specified by the instructor.

Note: This procedure will be performed on a radiographic-type mannikin.

Time limit: _____ Other conditions: _____

Points per step = _____ Maximum score = _____ Passing score = _____

*Check the left box **only** if step is performed correctly.*
Place score in the adjacent box. .

	Evaluator #1	Evaluator #2
1. Gathered and prepared appropriate supplies.	☐ ☐	☐ ☐
2. Seated the patient, placed the lead apron and thyroid collar, and explained the procedure.	☐ ☐	☐ ☐
3. Positioned the patient appropriately for each exposure.	☐ ☐	☐ ☐
4. Adjusted control panel settings appropriately for each exposure.	☐ ☐	☐ ☐
5. Positioned the film and PID appropriately for each exposure.	☐ ☐	☐ ☐
6. Exposed the prescribed number and type of films.	☐ ☐	☐ ☐
7. Followed the appropriate exposure control measures throughout the procedure.	☐ ☐	☐ ☐
8. Transported the exposed films to processing area.	☐ ☐	☐ ☐

Student's score _____ _____

Evaluator's comments

Evaluation Form

Competency 17 - 2 *Processing and Mounting Radiographs*

Performance Objective: The student will process and mount a series of dental radiographs that are free of processing errors.

Note: The instructor will indicate whether automatic or manual processing equipment is to be used.

Time limit: _____	Other conditions: _____
Points per step = _____	Maximum score = _____	Passing score = _____

*Check the left box **only** if step is performed correctly.*
Place score in the adjacent box.

	Evaluator #1	Evaluator #2
1. Assembled supplies and prepared work area.	☐ ☐	☐ ☐
2. Identified films with the patient's name and the date throughout processing and mounting.	☐ ☐	☐ ☐
3. Processed exposed films appropriately for the method being used.	☐ ☐	☐ ☐
4. Discarded contaminated film packets and lead foil in an appropriate manner.	☐ ☐	☐ ☐
5. Films were free of processing errors.	☐ ☐	☐ ☐
6. Left the processing area clean and ready for reuse.	☐ ☐	☐ ☐
7. Placed identification on film mount.	☐ ☐	☐ ☐
8. Placed radiographs in the appropriate windows of the radiographic mount.	☐ ☐	☐ ☐
9. Followed the appropriate exposure control measures throughout the procedure.	☐ ☐	☐ ☐

Student's score   _____   _____

Evaluator's comments

Evaluation Form

Competency 17 - 3 *Evaluating Radiographs for Diagnostic Quality*

Performance Objective: The student will evaluate the series for diagnostic quality and determine the number of retakes required.

> *Time limit:* _____ *Other conditions:* _____
>
> *Points per step =* _____ *Maximum score =* _____ *Passing score =* _____

*Check the left box **only** if step is performed correctly.*
Place score in the adjacent box.

	Evaluator #1	Evaluator #2
1. Placed mounted survey on view box.	☐ ☐	☐ ☐
2. Determined that the entire length of each tooth is visible and dimensionally accurate in at least one view.	☐ ☐	☐ ☐
3. Determined that the apex of the roots of each tooth are visible in at least one view.	☐ ☐	☐ ☐
4. Determined that 2 to 3 mm of surrounding tissues are visible in at least one view.	☐ ☐	☐ ☐
5. Determined that each interproximal contact area is open in at least one view.	☐ ☐	☐ ☐
6. Determined that contrast and density are adequate to show the details of the structures clearly.	☐ ☐	☐ ☐
7. Identified number and position of retakes required.	☐ ☐	☐ ☐
8. Stated the cause of each error and identified the action required to prevent a recurrence of that error.	☐ ☐	☐ ☐

Student's score   _____   _____

Evaluator's comments

Evaluation Form

Competency 18 - 1 Obtaining Patient Health History Information

Performance Objective: Given a health history form, the student will aid a "patient" (another student) in completing the form. (To protect privacy, the student serving as the patient can make up a health history for this exercise.)

Important: *The instructor will provide the student with a health history form.*

Time limit: _____ Other conditions: _____

Points per step = _____ Maximum score = _____ Passing score = _____

Check the left box **only** if step is performed correctly.
Place score in the adjacent box.

	Evaluator #1	Evaluator #2
1. Explained to the patient the purpose of the form and emphasized the importance of answering all questions.	☐ ☐	☐ ☐
2. Gave the patient the form and a pen or pencil.	☐ ☐	☐ ☐
3. Gave the patient adequate time to complete the form.	☐ ☐	☐ ☐
4. Reviewed the completed form to determine that all questions had been answered.	☐ ☐	☐ ☐
5. Encouraged the patient to answer any remaining questions.	☐ ☐	☐ ☐
6. If applicable, informed the dentist of any difficulties or questions regarding the questionnaire.	☐ ☐	☐ ☐
7. Followed up on any "yes" or ambiguous answers.	☐ ☐	☐ ☐
8. Thanked the patient for his or her cooperation.	☐ ☐	☐ ☐

Student's score _____ _____

Evaluator's comments

Evaluation Form

Competency 18 - 2 *Recording a Dental Examination*

Performance Objective: Given a dental chart tooth diagram, the student will demonstrate recording the charting findings as dictated by the instructor.

Important: *The instructor will supply the student with a dental chart tooth diagram. The instructor will dictate an examination consisting of 10 items to be recorded on the diagram.*

Time limit: _____ Other conditions: _____

Points per step = _____ Maximum score = _____ Passing score = _____

*Check the left box **only** if step is performed correctly.*
Place score in the adjacent box.

	Evaluator #1	Evaluator #2
1. Recorded item #1 correctly.	☐ ☐	☐ ☐
2. Recorded item #2 correctly.	☐ ☐	☐ ☐
3. Recorded item #3 correctly.	☐ ☐	☐ ☐
4. Recorded item #4 correctly.	☐ ☐	☐ ☐
5. Recorded item #5 correctly.	☐ ☐	☐ ☐
6. Recorded item #6 correctly.	☐ ☐	☐ ☐
7. Recorded item #7 correctly.	☐ ☐	☐ ☐
8. Recorded item #8 correctly.	☐ ☐	☐ ☐
9. Recorded item #9 correctly.	☐ ☐	☐ ☐
10. Recorded item #10 correctly.	☐ ☐	☐ ☐

Student's score   _____   _____

Evaluator's comments

SEXTANT SCORE

MONTH   DAY   YEAR

Evaluation Form

Competency 18 - 3 *Recording PSR scores*

Performance Objective: Using the diagram above, the student will record PSR scores by sextant as dictated by the instructor.

Important: *The instructor will dictate a score for each of the sextants.*

Time limit: _____ *Other conditions:* _____

Points per step = _____ *Maximum score* = _____ *Passing score* = _____

*Check the left box **only** if step is performed correctly.*
Place score in the adjacent box.

                                             Evaluator #1   Evaluator #2

1. Recorded sextant 1 correctly.   ☐ ☐   ☐ ☐

2. Recorded sextant 2 correctly.   ☐ ☐   ☐ ☐

3. Recorded sextant 3 correctly.   ☐ ☐   ☐ ☐

4. Recorded sextant 4 correctly.   ☐ ☐   ☐ ☐

5. Recorded sextant 5 correctly.   ☐ ☐   ☐ ☐

6. Recorded sextant 6 correctly.   ☐ ☐   ☐ ☐

Student's score   _____   _____

Evaluator's comments

Date	Tooth	Service Rendered

Evaluation Form

Competency 18 - 4 *Recording Dental Treatment*

Performance Objective: Using the form shown above, the student will use the abbreviations taught in class to record treatment as dictated by the instructor.

Important: *The instructor should prepare a description of treatment that includes at least 5 items that must be included in the treatment record. This information is dictated to the students.*

Time limit: _____ Other conditions: _____

Points per step = _____ Maximum score = _____ Passing score = _____

*Check the left box **only** if step is performed correctly.*
Place score in the adjacent box.

		Evaluator #1	Evaluator #2
1.	Recorded treatment item #1 correctly.	☐ ☐	☐ ☐
2.	Recorded treatment item #2 correctly.	☐ ☐	☐ ☐
3.	Recorded treatment item #3 correctly.	☐ ☐	☐ ☐
4.	Recorded treatment item #4 correctly.	☐ ☐	☐ ☐
5.	Recorded treatment item #5 correctly.	☐ ☐	☐ ☐

Student's score _____ _____

Evaluator's comments

Evaluation Form

Competency 19 - 1 *Obtaining Alginate Impressions*

Performance Objective: The student will obtain diagnostic quality alginate impressions of the mandibular and maxillary arches.

Time limit: _____ Other conditions: _____

Points per step = _____ Maximum score = _____ Passing score = _____

*Check the left box **only** if step is performed correctly.*
Place score in the adjacent box.

	Evaluator #1	Evaluator #2
1. Gathered appropriate supplies.	☐ ☐	☐ ☐
2. Draped the seated patient and explained the procedure.	☐ ☐	☐ ☐
3. Asked patient to take out any removable prosthesis.	☐ ☐	☐ ☐
4. Used air-water syringe and HVE to rinse patient's mouth.	☐ ☐	☐ ☐
5. Selected and modified the appropriate trays.	☐ ☐	☐ ☐

Mandibular impression:

6. Mixed impression material and loaded tray.	☐ ☐	☐ ☐
7. Placed the loaded tray into patient's mouth and seated the tray properly.	☐ ☐	☐ ☐
8. Removed tray when material was set. Used air-water syringe and HVE to rinse patient's mouth.	☐ ☐	☐ ☐

Maxillary impression:

9. Mixed impression material and loaded tray.	☐ ☐	☐ ☐
10. Placed the loaded tray into patient's mouth and seated the tray properly.	☐ ☐	☐ ☐
11. Removed tray when material was set. Used air-water syringe and HVE to rinse patient's mouth.	☐ ☐	☐ ☐
12. Prepared supplies for disinfection or sterilization and return to storage.	☐ ☐	☐ ☐
13. Followed the appropriate exposure control measures throughout the procedure.	☐ ☐	☐ ☐

Student's score _____ _____

Evaluator's comments

Evaluation Form

Competency 19 - 2 *Evaluating Mandibular and Maxillary Alginate Impressions*

Performance Objective: The student will evaluate the mandibular and maxillary impressions to determine that they are adequate to produce casts of diagnostic quality.

Time limit: _____ *Other conditions:* _____

Points per step = _____ *Maximum score* = _____ *Passing score* = _____

---

*Check the left box **only** if step is performed correctly.*
Place score in the adjacent box.

	Evaluator #1	Evaluator #2

Evaluating the mandibular impression:

1. The impression shows that the tray was centered in patient's mouth. ☐ ☐   ☐ ☐

2. In critical areas, the impression material was smooth and free of voids. ☐ ☐   ☐ ☐

3. The retromolar pad was recorded in the impression. ☐ ☐   ☐ ☐

4. The peripheral roll was adequate. ☐ ☐   ☐ ☐

5. Each frenum was represented. ☐ ☐   ☐ ☐

6. The impression was acceptable. ☐ ☐   ☐ ☐

Evaluating the maxillary impression:

7. The impression shows that the tray was centered in the patient's mouth. ☐ ☐   ☐ ☐

8. In critical areas, the impression material was smooth and free of voids. ☐ ☐   ☐ ☐

9. The tuberosity was recorded in the impression. ☐ ☐   ☐ ☐

10. The peripheral roll was adequate. ☐ ☐   ☐ ☐

11. Each frenum was represented. ☐ ☐   ☐ ☐

12. The impression was acceptable. ☐ ☐   ☐ ☐

Student's score _____   _____

Evaluator's comments

Evaluation Form

Competency 19 - 3 *Obtaining a Wax-Bite Registration*

Performance Objective: The student will obtain an acceptable wax bite registration. This procedure will be performed with a minimum of patient discomfort.

Time limit: _____	*Other conditions:* _____
Points per step = _____	*Maximum score* = _____ *Passing score* = _____

*Check the left box **only** if step is performed correctly.*
Place score in the adjacent box.

	Evaluator #1	Evaluator #2
1. Gathered appropriate supplies.	☐ ☐	☐ ☐
2. Provided appropriate patient instruction.	☐ ☐	☐ ☐
3. Prepared material appropriately.	☐ ☐	☐ ☐
4. Placed softened wax on occlusal surfaces of the mandibular teeth.	☐ ☐	☐ ☐
5. Instructed patient to close his teeth into the wax.	☐ ☐	☐ ☐
6. Instructed patient to open his mouth and removed wax.	☐ ☐	☐ ☐

Evaluated bite registration for adequacy:

	Evaluator #1	Evaluator #2
7. Patient did not bite through wax.	☐ ☐	☐ ☐
8. Patient bit hard enough to record occlusal surfaces.	☐ ☐	☐ ☐
9. Bite registration was acceptable.	☐ ☐	☐ ☐
10. Followed appropriate exposure control measures throughout the procedure	☐ ☐	☐ ☐

Student's score   _____   _____

Evaluator's comments

Evaluation Form

Competency 19 - 4 *Producing Diagnostic Casts in Plaster*

Performance Objective: The student will use the pouring procedure specified by the instructor to produce diagnostic casts in plaster. The wax bite will be used to articulate the casts as they are trimmed to an acceptable appearance.

Note: Criteria for acceptable appearance will be determined by the instructor.

Time limit: _____ *Other conditions:* _____

Points per step = _____ *Maximum score =* _____ *Passing score =* _____

---

*Check the left box **only** if step is performed correctly.*
Place score in the adjacent box.   Evaluator #1   Evaluator #2

1. Gathered appropriate supplies.   ☐ ☐   ☐ ☐

2. Gently removed excess water from the impressions.   ☐ ☐   ☐ ☐

3. Prepared a mix of plaster and poured each of the
   impressions.   ☐ ☐   ☐ ☐

4. When the plaster had set, separated the impressions
   and cast without damage to the cast.   ☐ ☐   ☐ ☐

5. Evaluated casts for diagnostic quality and determined
   that casts were free of voids in critical areas.   ☐ ☐   ☐ ☐

6. Put on face shield or safety goggles, then used model
   trimmer to trim the casts to be esthetically acceptable.   ☐ ☐   ☐ ☐

7. Placed patient identification on the casts.   ☐ ☐   ☐ ☐

8. Left equipment and work area ready for reuse.   ☐ ☐   ☐ ☐

Student's score   _____   _____

Evaluator's comments

Evaluation Form

Competency 20 - 1 *Applying Topical Anesthetic*

Performance Objective: The student will gather the necessary equipment and then demonstrate the application of a topical anesthetic ointment in preparation for the injection of local anesthetic solution for the maxillary left central incisor.

Time limit: _____ Other conditions: _____

Points per step = _____ Maximum score = _____ Passing score = _____

Check the left box **only** if step is performed correctly.
Place score in the adjacent box.

	Evaluator #1	Evaluator #2
1. Gathered appropriate supplies.	☐ ☐	☐ ☐
2. Explained procedure to patient.	☐ ☐	☐ ☐
3. Placed an appropriate amount of topical anesthetic ointment on cotton-tipped applicator.	☐ ☐	☐ ☐
4. Used a sterile gauze sponge to gently dry the correct injection site.	☐ ☐	☐ ☐
5. Removed gauze sponge. Positioned the applicator with the ointment directly on the injection site.	☐ ☐	☐ ☐
6. Removed applicator after time recommended by the ointment manufacturer.	☐ ☐	☐ ☐
7. Checked the comfort of the patient until the operator was ready to begin the procedure.	☐ ☐	☐ ☐
8. Followed the appropriate exposure control measures throughout the procedure.	☐ ☐	☐ ☐

Student's score _____ _____

Evaluator's comments

Evaluation Form

Competency 20 - 2 *Preparing a Local Anesthetic Syringe*

Performance Objective: The student will demonstrate the preparation of a local anesthetic syringe for an infiltration injection of anesthetic solution using an aspirating syringe and local anesthetic cartridge. The epinephrine ratio is specified by the dentist or instructor.

Time limit: _____ Other conditions: _____

Points per step = _____ Maximum score = _____ Passing score = _____

*Check the left box **only** if step is performed correctly.*
Place score in the adjacent box.

	Evaluator #1	Evaluator #2
1. Gathered appropriate supplies.	☐ ☐	☐ ☐
2. Disinfected needle end of anesthetic cartridge.	☐ ☐	☐ ☐
3. Placed cartridge in syringe and engaged harpoon.	☐ ☐	☐ ☐
4. Opened disposable needle packet without touching or contaminating the needle.	☐ ☐	☐ ☐
5. Attached the needle to the syringe.	☐ ☐	☐ ☐
6. Loosened the needle guard, but left it on the needle.	☐ ☐	☐ ☐
7. Placed prepared syringe on the instrument tray out of the patient's sight.	☐ ☐	☐ ☐
8. Followed the appropriate exposure control measures throughout the procedure.	☐ ☐	☐ ☐

Student's score _____ _____

Evaluator's comments

Evaluation Form

Competency 20 - 3 *Caring for a Used Local Anesthetic Syringe*

Performance Objective: The student will demonstrate safely disassembling a used local anesthetic syringe in preparation for sterilization.

Time limit: _____ *Other conditions:* _____

Points per step = _____ *Maximum score =* _____ *Passing score =* _____

Check the left box **only** *if step is performed correctly.*
Place score in the adjacent box.

		Evaluator #1		Evaluator #2	
1. Was still gloved from previous procedure.		☐	☐	☐	☐
2. Recapped needle using a one-handed or needle holder technique.		☐	☐	☐	☐
3. Removed needle and discarded appropriately.		☐	☐	☐	☐
4. Removed the used anesthetic cartridge and discarded appropriately.		☐	☐	☐	☐
5. Placed the syringe on the instrument tray to be returned to the sterilization center.		☐	☐	☐	☐

Student's score   _____   _____

Evaluator's comments

Evaluation Form

Competency 21 - 1 *Coronal Polishing on a Typodont*

Performance Objective: The student will demonstrate coronal polishing technique on a typodont or mannikin.

Note: In states where coronal polishing is legal, under proper supervision, the student will eventually perform this procedure on a patient. In other states, the student should be prepared to assist during a coronal polishing procedure.

Time limit: _____ *Other conditions:* _____

Points per step = _____ *Maximum score =* _____ *Passing score =* _____

*Check the left box **only** if step is performed correctly.*
Place score in the adjacent box.

	Evaluator #1	Evaluator #2
1. Gathered appropriate supplies.	☐ ☐	☐ ☐
2. Positioned typodont correctly for each quadrant.	☐ ☐	☐ ☐
3. Maintained correct operator position and posture for each quadrant.	☐ ☐	☐ ☐
4. Demonstrated use of mouth mirror for retraction.	☐ ☐	☐ ☐
5. Demonstrated use of mouth mirror for reflection of light.	☐ ☐	☐ ☐
6. Maintained adequate fulcrum positions for each quadrant.	☐ ☐	☐ ☐
7. Applied appropriate amount of polishing agent.	☐ ☐	☐ ☐
8. Utilized a "pat and wipe" polishing stroke.	☐ ☐	☐ ☐
9. Controlled handpiece speed and pressure throughout.	☐ ☐	☐ ☐
10. Followed the appropriate exposure control measures throughout the procedure.	☐ ☐	☐ ☐

Student's score _____ _____

Evaluator's comments

Evaluation Form

Competency 22 - 1 *Punching Dental Dam for Maxillary Anterior
and Mandibular Posterior Placement*

Performance Objective: The student will demonstrate punching two dental dams, one for maxillary anterior placement and one for mandibular posterior placement.

Note: The teeth to be exposed will be specified by the instructor.

Time limit: _____   Other conditions: _____

Points per step = _____   Maximum score = _____   Passing score = _____

*Check the left box **only** if step is performed correctly.
Place score in the adjacent box.*

	Evaluator #1	Evaluator #2
1. Gathered appropriate supplies.	☐ ☐	☐ ☐
2. Marked specified holes for maxillary anterior placement.	☐ ☐	☐ ☐
3. Punched holes for maxillary anterior placement.	☐ ☐	☐ ☐

Evaluated maxillary dam preparation:

	Evaluator #1	Evaluator #2
4. Holes were appropriately sized.	☐ ☐	☐ ☐
5. Holes were appropriately spaced and positioned.	☐ ☐	☐ ☐
6. Holes were punched cleanly without ragged edges.	☐ ☐	☐ ☐
7. Marked specified holes for mandibular posterior placement. ·	☐ ☐	☐ ☐
8. Punched holes for mandibular posterior placement.	☐ ☐	☐ ☐

Evaluated mandibular dam preparation:

	Evaluator #1	Evaluator #2
9. Holes were appropriately sized.	☐ ☐	☐ ☐
10. Holes were appropriately spaced and positioned.	☐ ☐	☐ ☐
11. Holes were punched cleanly without ragged edges.	☐ ☐	☐ ☐
12. Followed the appropriate exposure control measures throughout the procedure.	☐ ☐	☐ ☐

Student's score   _____   _____

Evaluator's comments

63

Evaluation Form

Competency 22 - 2 *Assisting in Dental Dam Placement*

Performance Objective: The student will assist the operator in the placement of the dental dam. (A mannikin may be used for this demonstration; however, appropriate exposure control protocols must be followed.)

Time limit: _____	*Other conditions:* _____
Points per step = _____	*Maximum score* = _____ *Passing score* = _____

*Check the left box **only** if step is performed correctly.*
Place score in the adjacent box.

	Evaluator #1	Evaluator #2
1. Prepared appropriate supplies.	☐ ☐	☐ ☐
2. Prepared clamp with a floss ligature.	☐ ☐	☐ ☐
3. Placed clamp in dental dam forceps. Passed forceps to the operator in the position of use.	☐ ☐	☐ ☐
4. Received clamp and forceps. Passed the clamp bow through the keyhole of the dam.	☐ ☐	☐ ☐
5. Returned clamp, forceps, and dam to operator.	☐ ☐	☐ ☐
6. Received forceps. Passed dental dam frame to the operator.	☐ ☐	☐ ☐
7. Aided operator in passing dam between proximal contacts.	☐ ☐	☐ ☐
8. Aided operator in inverting dental dam.	☐ ☐	☐ ☐
9. Aided operator in ligating and stabilizing dental dam.	☐ ☐	☐ ☐
10. Followed the appropriate exposure control measures throughout the procedure.	☐ ☐	☐ ☐

Student's score _____   _____

Evaluator's comments

Evaluation Form

Competency 22 - 3 *Assisting in Dental Dam Removal*

Performance Objective: The student will demonstrate assisting the operator in the removal of dental dam. (A mannikin may be used for this demonstration; however, appropriate exposure control protocols must be followed.)

Time limit: _____	*Other conditions:* _____
Points per step = _____	*Maximum score =* _____ *Passing score =* _____

*Check the left box **only** if step is performed correctly.*
Place score in the adjacent box.

	Evaluator #1	Evaluator #2
1. Had prepared appropriate supplies.	☐ ☐	☐ ☐
2. Passed instrument to cut and remove ligatures.	☐ ☐	☐ ☐
3. Received used instrument. Passed suture scissors to cut each dental dam septum.	☐ ☐	☐ ☐
4. Received suture scissors. Passed dental dam clamp forceps.	☐ ☐	☐ ☐
5. Received dental dam clamp forceps and clamp. Received dental dam frame and used dental dam.	☐ ☐	☐ ☐
6. Checked dental dam for tears or missing pieces.	☐ ☐	☐ ☐
7. Reported status of used dental dam to the operator.	☐ ☐	☐ ☐
8. Used tissue to gently wipe patient's face clean.	☐ ☐	☐ ☐
9. Used the air-water syringe and HVE tip to rinse the patient's mouth.	☐ ☐	☐ ☐
10. Followed the appropriate exposure control measures throughout the procedure.	☐ ☐	☐ ☐

Student's score   _____   _____

Evaluator's comments

Evaluation Form

Competency 23 - 1 *Mixing Zinc Phosphate for Cementation*

Performance Objective: The student will assemble the necessary equipment and materials, then correctly manipulate the material for use in the cementation of a cast crown.

Note:. If a crown is available, the student will also be asked to place the cement inside the crown.

Time limit: _____ *Other conditions:* _____

Points per step = _____ *Maximum score* = _____ *Passing score* = _____

---

*Check the left box **only** if step is performed correctly.*
Place score in the adjacent box.

	Evaluator #1	Evaluator #2
1. Gathered appropriate supplies.	☐ ☐	☐ ☐
2. Read manufacturer's directions.	☐ ☐	☐ ☐
3. Dispensed materials in the proper sequence and immediately recapped the containers.	☐ ☐	☐ ☐
4. Incorporated powder into the liquid according to the manufacturer's directions.	☐ ☐	☐ ☐
5. Completed the mix within the appropriate working time.	☐ ☐	☐ ☐
6. Tested mass for droplet break 1 inch from slab.	☐ ☐	☐ ☐
7. *Optional:* Filled the crown with cement.	☐ ☐	☐ ☐
8. When finished, cleaned slab and spatula in preparation for sterilization.	☐ ☐	☐ ☐
9. Returned supplies to storage or sterilization center.	☐ ☐	☐ ☐
10. Followed the appropriate exposure control measures throughout the procedure.	☐ ☐	☐ ☐

Student's score   _____   _____

Evaluator's comments

Evaluation Form

Competency 23 - 2 *Mixing Zinc Oxide-Eugenol for a Sedative Base*

Performance Objective: The student will assemble the necessary equipment and materials, then correctly manipulate the material for use as a sedative base.

Time limit: _____ *Other conditions:* _____

Points per step = _____ *Maximum score =* _____ *Passing score =* _____

---

*Check the left box **only** if step is performed correctly.*
Place score in the adjacent box.

	Evaluator #1	Evaluator #2
1. Gathered appropriate supplies.	❑ ❑	❑ ❑
2. Read manufacturer's directions.	❑ ❑	❑ ❑
3. Dispensed materials in appropriate amounts.	❑ ❑	❑ ❑
4. Appropriately recapped containers immediately after use.	❑ ❑	❑ ❑
5. Incorporated the powder and liquid according to the manufacturer's directions.	❑ ❑	❑ ❑
6. Completed the mix to the proper thickness within the appropriate working time.	❑ ❑	❑ ❑
7. When finished, cared for equipment in preparation for sterilization.	❑ ❑	❑ ❑
8. Returned supplies to storage or sterilization center.	❑ ❑	❑ ❑
9. Followed the appropriate exposure control measures throughout the procedure.	❑ ❑	❑ ❑

Student's score _____ _____

Evaluator's comments

Evaluation Form

Competency 24 - 1 *Constructing a Custom Impression Tray*

Performance Objective: The student will construct a full arch custom tray for a mandibular impression using acrylic resin tray material and wax spacing material.

Time limit: _____	Other conditions: _____
Points per step = _____	Maximum score = _____ Passing score = _____

Check the left box only if step is performed correctly.
Place score in the adjacent box.

                                                                      Evaluator #1   Evaluator #2

1. Gathered the appropriate supplies. ☐ ☐   ☐ ☐

2. Evaluated the cast and eliminated defects that would impair placement or removal of the tray. ☐ ☐   ☐ ☐

3. Placed the spacer. ☐ ☐   ☐ ☐

4. Prepared the stops. ☐ ☐   ☐ ☐

5. Painted the spacer and surrounding area with separating medium. ☐ ☐   ☐ ☐

6. Mixed and placed the tray material. ☐ ☐   ☐ ☐

7. Prepared and placed the tray handle. ☐ ☐   ☐ ☐

8. After the initial set, removed the spacer and replaced the tray on the cast to complete the set. ☐ ☐   ☐ ☐

Evaluated the completed tray for acceptability:

9. The tray covered the desired area. ☐ ☐   ☐ ☐

10. The stops were properly positioned. ☐ ☐   ☐ ☐

11. The handle was appropriately placed. ☐ ☐   ☐ ☐

12. Smoothed edges of tray as necessary. ☐ ☐   ☐ ☐

13. Painted interior of tray with the appropriate adhesive. ☐ ☐   ☐ ☐

Student's score   _____   _____

Evaluator's comments

Evaluation Form

Competency 24 - 2 *Mixing Syringe-Type and*
Tray-Type Impression Materials

Performance Objective: The student will follow the manufacturer's instructions for mixing the impression materials selected by the instructor. The custom tray fabricated by the student may be used in this procedure.

Note: The instructor will select the type of impression materials to be mixed.

Time limit: _____ Other conditions: _____

Points per step = _____ Maximum score = _____ Passing score = _____

*Check the left box **only** if step is performed correctly.*
Place score in the adjacent box.

	Evaluator #1	Evaluator #2
1. Gathered the appropriate supplies.	☐ ☐	☐ ☐
2. Followed the manufacturer's directions for dispensing and mixing the syringe-type material.	☐ ☐	☐ ☐
3. If applicable, loaded and passed the impression syringe.	☐ ☐	☐ ☐
4. Followed the manufacturer's directions for dispensing and mixing the tray-type material.	☐ ☐	☐ ☐
5. Loaded and passed the impression tray.	☐ ☐	☐ ☐
6. Described how the completed impression would be disinfected.	☐ ☐	☐ ☐
7. Prepared supplies and equipment to be returned to the sterilization center.	☐ ☐	☐ ☐
8. Followed the appropriate exposure control measures throughout the procedure.	☐ ☐	☐ ☐

Student's score   _____   _____

Evaluator's comments

Evaluation Form

Competency 24 - 3 *Assisting in a Two-Step Impression Technique*

Performance Objective: The student will prepare the impression materials and care for the impression during a two-step technique using silicone impression materials.

Note: A typodont will be used to simulate taking the preliminary impression.

Time limit: _____ Other conditions: _____

Points per step = _____ Maximum score = _____ Passing score = _____

*Check the left box **only** if step is performed correctly.*
Place score in the adjacent box.

	Evaluator #1		Evaluator #2	
1. Gathered the appropriate supplies including an impression tray painted with adhesive.	☐	☐	☐	☐
2. Mixed putty base according to the manufacturer's directions.	☐	☐	☐	☐
3. Loaded the putty into the impression tray.	☐	☐	☐	☐
4. Placed an indentation in impression material where the teeth will be.	☐	☐	☐	☐
5. Placed plastic sheet spacer over impression material.	☐	☐	☐	☐
6. Passed the tray to the operator or placed the tray on the typodont.	☐	☐	☐	☐
7. Removed the spacer from the impression and checked for defects (large bubbles or wrinkles).	☐	☐	☐	☐
8. Used a scalpel to trim away undercuts in the impression.	☐	☐	☐	☐
9. Cared for the impression appropriately until time to take the second impression.	☐	☐	☐	☐
10. Described preparation of the extruder gun with wash and the steps in the final impression.	☐	☐	☐	☐
11. Cared for the completed impression appropriately.	☐	☐	☐	☐
12. Prepared supplies and equipment to be returned to the sterilization center.	☐	☐	☐	☐
13. Followed the appropriate exposure control measures throughout the procedure.	☐	☐	☐	☐

Student's score _____ _____

Evaluator's comments

Evaluation Form

Competency 25 - 1 *Assisting in the Placement of an Amalgam Restoration*

Performance Objective: The student will demonstrate the role of the chairside assistant throughout all steps in the preparation, placement, and finishing of a Class II amalgam restoration

Note: The treatment area has been cleaned and protective barriers are in place. All supplies are in place and the patient has been seated and positioned. Local anesthetic has been administered. (The operator did not elect to use dental dam.)

Time limit: _____ Other Conditions: _____

Points per step = _____ Maximum score = _____ Passing score = _____

Check the left box **only** if step is performed correctly.
Place score in the adjacent box.   Evaluator #1   Evaluator #2

1. Anticipated operator's needs and demonstrated effective and appropriate use of the HVE and air-water syringe. ☐ ☐   ☐ ☐

2. Anticipated operator's needs and demonstrated effective and appropriate soft tissue retraction. ☐ ☐   ☐ ☐

3. Anticipated operator's needs and demonstrated effective and appropriate exchange of instruments and materials. ☐ ☐   ☐ ☐

4. Mixed and passed (or placed) cavity liner and base in appropriate quantity and sequence. ☐ ☐   ☐ ☐

5. Assembled, passed, or placed matrix band and wedge. ☐ ☐   ☐ ☐

6. Mixed amalgam and loaded amalgam carriers. ☐ ☐   ☐ ☐

7. Exchanged amalgam carriers and condensers as needed. ☐ ☐   ☐ ☐

8. Assisted in matrix removal and passed carving instruments. ☐ ☐   ☐ ☐

9. Passed (or placed) articulating paper and passed carvers as needed. ☐ ☐   ☐ ☐

10. Rinsed patient's mouth to remove debris and excess water. ☐ ☐   ☐ ☐

11. Anticipated operator's needs throughout. ☐ ☐   ☐ ☐

12. Followed the appropriate exposure control measures throughout the procedure. ☐ ☐   ☐ ☐

Student's score   _____   _____

Evaluator's comments

71

Evaluation Form

Competency 25 - 2 *Assisting in the Placement of a Composite Restoration*

Performance Objective: The student will demonstrate the role of the chairside assistant throughout all steps in the preparation, placement, and finishing of a Class III light-cured composite restoration

Note: The treatment area has been cleaned and protective barriers are in place. All supplies are in place and the patient has been seated and positioned. No local anesthetic is required. (The operator did not elect to use dental dam.) No liner or base is required.

> *Time limit:* _____ *Other Conditions:* _____
>
> *Points per step* = _____ *Maximum score* = _____ *Passing score* = _____

*Check the left box **only** if step is performed correctly.*
Place score in the adjacent box.

	Evaluator #1	Evaluator #2
1. Anticipated operator's needs and demonstrated effective and appropriate use of the HVE and air-water syringe.	☐ ☐	☐ ☐
2. Anticipated operator's needs and demonstrated effective and appropriate soft tissue retraction.	☐ ☐	☐ ☐
3. Anticipated operator's needs and demonstrated effective and appropriate exchange of instruments and materials.	☐ ☐	☐ ☐
4. Assisted in placement of the matrix.	☐ ☐	☐ ☐
5. Anticipated and demonstrated appropriate help during the etching procedure and application of bonding agent.	☐ ☐	☐ ☐
6. Passed composite of the appropriate shade.	☐ ☐	☐ ☐
7. Passed or held the curing light as directed.	☐ ☐	☐ ☐
8. Assisted in removing matrix.	☐ ☐	☐ ☐
9. Prepared and passed handpiece and/or hand instruments for finishing restoration.	☐ ☐	☐ ☐
10. Rinsed patient's mouth to remove debris and excess water.	☐ ☐	☐ ☐
11. Anticipated operator's needs throughout.	☐ ☐	☐ ☐
12. Followed the appropriate exposure control measures throughout the procedure.	☐ ☐	☐ ☐

Student's score   _____   _____

Evaluator's comments

Evaluation Form

Competency 26 - 1 *Assisting During Periodontal Surgery*

Performance Objective: Given an appropriate selection of periodontal surgical instruments, the student will select the instruments and materials required for the surgical procedure specified by the instructor.

Note: The instructor will specify the type of surgery to be performed and the instruments to be included on the preset tray. The instructor will then role play the dentist performing that surgery. Another student will act as the patient.

Time limit: _____ Other Conditions: _____

Points per step = _____ Maximum score = _____ Passing score = _____

*Check the left box **only** if step is performed correctly.*
Place score in the adjacent box.

	Evaluator #1	Evaluator #2
1. Gathered the appropriate supplies as specified for the procedure.	☐ ☐	☐ ☐
2. Arranged the instruments in the sequence of use.	☐ ☐	☐ ☐
3. Stated the use of each instrument.	☐ ☐	☐ ☐
4. Covered the tray to protect it until used.	☐ ☐	☐ ☐
5. Maintained sterile technique while preparing the tray.	☐ ☐	☐ ☐
6. Scrubbed hands and put on PPE in preparation for assisting during the procedure.	☐ ☐	☐ ☐
7. Maintained a clear operating field at all times.	☐ ☐	☐ ☐
8. Anticipated the dentist's needs throughout.	☐ ☐	☐ ☐
9. Maintained patient comfort.	☐ ☐	☐ ☐
10. Followed the appropriate exposure control measures throughout the procedure.	☐ ☐	☐ ☐

Student's score _____ _____

Evaluator's comments

Evaluation Form

Competency 26 - 2 *Preparing Periodontal Surgical Dressing*

Performance Objective: The student will demonstrate mixing noneugenol periodontal surgical dressing.

Note: The instructor will identify the location and extent of the surgical site.

Time limit: _____	*Other Conditions:* _____
Points per step = _____	*Maximum score* = _____ *Passing score* = _____

Check the left box **only** *if step is performed correctly.*
Place score in the adjacent box.

	Evaluator #1	Evaluator #2
1. Gathered appropriate supplies.	☐ ☐	☐ ☐
2. Read and followed the manufacturer's instructions.	☐ ☐	☐ ☐
3. Dispensed proper amount of material onto mixing pad.	☐ ☐	☐ ☐
4. Recapped tubes immediately.	☐ ☐	☐ ☐
5. Thoroughly mixed base and catalyst pastes.	☐ ☐	☐ ☐
6. Placed mixed material in cup of water.	☐ ☐	☐ ☐
7. Rolled material into correct length roll.	☐ ☐	☐ ☐
8. Prepared used supplies for return to the sterilization center.	☐ ☐	☐ ☐
9. Followed the appropriate exposure control measures throughout the procedure.	☐ ☐	☐ ☐

Student's score _____ _____

Evaluator's comments

Evaluation Form

Competency 27 - 1 *Applying Topical Fluoride Gel*

Performance Objective: The student will demonstrate application of a topical fluoride gel on a patient or typodont.

Note: An assistant is allowed to perform this function **only** in states where it is legal under the rules and regulations of the state dental practice act.

Time limit: _____ Other Conditions: _____

Points per step = _____ Maximum score = _____ Passing score = _____

Check the left box **only** if step is performed correctly.
Place score in the adjacent box.

	Evaluator #1	Evaluator #2
1. Gathered appropriate supplies.	☐ ☐	☐ ☐
2. Seated patient upright and explained the procedure. Cautioned the patient **not** to swallow the gel.	☐ ☐	☐ ☐
3. Selected the appropriate tray and lined it with fluoride gel.	☐ ☐	☐ ☐
4. Dried the teeth using air from the air-water syringe.	☐ ☐	☐ ☐
5. Inserted the tray and placed the saliva ejector.	☐ ☐	☐ ☐
6. Set timer for time specified by manufacturer's instructions.	☐ ☐	☐ ☐
7. Stayed with patient. Upon completion of the treatment removed the tray.	☐ ☐	☐ ☐
8. Used the HVE tip to remove excess solution from patient's mouth.	☐ ☐	☐ ☐
9. Maintained patient comfort throughout.	☐ ☐	☐ ☐
10. Gave the patient and parent or guardian post-treatment instructions.	☐ ☐	☐ ☐
11. Followed the appropriate exposure control measures throughout the procedure.	☐ ☐	☐ ☐

Student's score   _____   _____

Evaluator's comments

75

Evaluation Form

Competency 27 - 2 *Applying Pit and Fissure Sealants*

Performance Objective: The student will demonstrate etching the teeth, applying the sealant, and light-curing it. This is to be performed on one or more extracted molars or premolars that have been polished with a fluoride-free abrasive, then rinsed and dried.

Note: An assistant is allowed to perform this function **only** in states where it is specified in the state dental practice act.

Time limit: _____ Other Conditions: _____

Points per step = _____ Maximum score = _____ Passing score = _____

*Check the left box **only** if step is performed correctly. Place score in the adjacent box.*

	Evaluator #1	Evaluator #2
1. Gathered appropriate supplies.	☐ ☐	☐ ☐
2. Stated how teeth have already been polished, rinsed, and thoroughly dried.	☐ ☐	☐ ☐
3. Described the necessary steps to prevent contamination by moisture or saliva.	☐ ☐	☐ ☐
4. Placed the etchant on the appropriate surfaces for the time specified by the manufacturer.	☐ ☐	☐ ☐
5. Rinsed and dried the teeth.	☐ ☐	☐ ☐
6. Verified the appearance of the etched surface. If not satisfactory, etched surfaces again.	☐ ☐	☐ ☐
7. Placed the sealant on the etched surfaces.	☐ ☐	☐ ☐
8. Light-cured the material according to the manufacturer's directions.	☐ ☐	☐ ☐
9. Checked occlusion. Stated how necessary adjustments would be made.	☐ ☐	☐ ☐
10. Requested that the dentist (instructor) evaluate the completed procedure before the patient was dismissed.	☐ ☐	☐ ☐
11. Maintained patient comfort throughout.	☐ ☐	☐ ☐
12. Followed the appropriate exposure control measures throughout the procedure.	☐ ☐	☐ ☐

Student's score _____ _____

Evaluator's comments

Evaluation Form

Competency 28 - 1 *Placing and Removing Orthodontic Separators*

Performance Objective: Using a typodont, the student will demonstrate the placement and removal of elastomeric ring orthodontic separators in preparation for band placement of maxillary first molars.

Time limit: _____ Other conditions: _____

Points per step = _____ Maximum score = _____ Passing score = _____

Check the left box **only** *if step is performed correctly.*
Place score in the adjacent box.   Evaluator #1   Evaluator #2

1. Gathered appropriate supplies.   ☐ ☐   ☐ ☐

2. Explained the procedure to the patient.   ☐ ☐   ☐ ☐

3. Placed the separator over the beaks of separating pliers.   ☐ ☐   ☐ ☐

4. Opened the pliers to stretch the separator ring.   ☐ ☐   ☐ ☐

5. Gently forced the ring through the contacts with a
   seesaw motion.   ☐ ☐   ☐ ☐

6. Stated how long this type of separator may be left in place. ☐ ☐   ☐ ☐

7. Selected an orthodontic scaler for removal of the separator. ☐ ☐   ☐ ☐

8. Slipped the scaler tip into the doughnut-shaped separator.   ☐ ☐   ☐ ☐

9. Use slight pressure to remove the ring from under
   the contact.   ☐ ☐   ☐ ☐

10. Used an appropriate fulcrum throughout.   ☐ ☐   ☐ ☐

11. Maintained patient comfort throughout.   ☐ ☐   ☐ ☐

12. Followed the appropriate exposure control measures
    throughout the procedure.   ☐ ☐   ☐ ☐

Student's score   _____   _____

Evaluator's comments

Evaluation Form

Competency 28 - 2 *Assisting in the Cementation of Orthodontic Bands*

Performance Objective: The student will demonstrate assisting during this procedure by mixing the cement, loading, and passing the band.

Note: In states where it is legal, the student may also demonstrate removing excess cement from a typodont.

Time limit: _____ Other conditions: _____

Points per step = _____ Maximum score = _____ Passing score = _____

Check the left box **only** if step is performed correctly.
Place score in the adjacent box.

	Evaluator #1	Evaluator #2
1. Gathered appropriate supplies including chilled glass slab.	☐ ☐	☐ ☐
2. Placed preselected orthodontic band on masking tape.	☐ ☐	☐ ☐
3. Dispensed cement according to the manufacturer's directions.	☐ ☐	☐ ☐
4. Replaced covers on containers immediately.	☐ ☐	☐ ☐
5. Mixed cement according to the manufacturer's directions to the appropriate consistency.	☐ ☐	☐ ☐
6. Mix allowed adequate working time.	☐ ☐	☐ ☐
7. Loaded cement into the band and passed the band to the operator.	☐ ☐	☐ ☐
8. Passed the band seater to the operator.	☐ ☐	☐ ☐
9. *Optional:* Demonstrated removal of excess cement while maintaining an appropriate fulcrum throughout.	☐ ☐	☐ ☐
10. Anticipated the operator's needs throughout.	☐ ☐	☐ ☐
11. Prepared supplies to be returned to the sterilization area.	☐ ☐	☐ ☐
12. Followed the appropriate exposure control measures throughout the procedure.	☐ ☐	☐ ☐

Student's score   _____   _____

Evaluator's comments

Evaluation Form

Competency 29 - 1 *Obtaining an Electric Pulp Testing Reading*

Performance Objective: The student will demonstrate obtaining a pulp vitality test reading on a control tooth. A normal (vital) maxillary central incisor is suggested for this purpose.

Time limit: _____ Other conditions: _____

Points per step = _____ Maximum score = _____ Passing score = _____

Check the left box **only** if step is performed correctly.
Place score in the adjacent box.

	Evaluator #1	Evaluator #2
1. Gathered appropriate supplies.	☐ ☐	☐ ☐
2. Explained the procedure to the patient.	☐ ☐	☐ ☐
3. Isolated the tooth to be tested and dried it thoroughly.	☐ ☐	☐ ☐
4. Placed a small dab of toothpaste on the tip of the pulp tester electrode.	☐ ☐	☐ ☐
5. Placed the tip of the electrode on the gingival one-third of the facial surface of the tooth to be tested.	☐ ☐	☐ ☐
6. Started with the setting at zero and gradually increased the setting until the patient responded.	☐ ☐	☐ ☐
7. Stopped as soon as the patient responded.	☐ ☐	☐ ☐
8. Recorded the reading on the patient's chart.	☐ ☐	☐ ☐
9. Maintained patient comfort through the procedure.	☐ ☐	☐ ☐
10. When finished, prepared supplies for sterilization or return to storage.	☐ ☐	☐ ☐
11. Followed the appropriate exposure control measures throughout the procedure.	☐ ☐	☐ ☐

Student's score _____ _____

Evaluator's comments

Evaluation Form

Competency 30 - 1 *Identifying Oral Surgery Instruments*

Performance Objective: Given an assortment of commonly used oral surgery instruments, the student will identify the instruments by type.

Important: *The instructor will select 10 commonly used surgery instruments (of different types) and number them 1 through 10.*

Time limit: _____ Other conditions: _____

Points per step = _____ Maximum score = _____ Passing score = _____

*Check the left box **only** if step is performed correctly. Place score in the adjacent box.*

	Evaluator #1	Evaluator #2
1. Correctly identified instrument #1 as a/an _____.	☐ ☐	☐ ☐
2. Correctly identified instrument #2 as a/an _____.	☐ ☐	☐ ☐
3. Correctly identified instrument #3 as a/an _____.	☐ ☐	☐ ☐
4. Correctly identified instrument #4 as a/an _____.	☐ ☐	☐ ☐
5. Correctly identified instrument #5 as a/an _____.	☐ ☐	☐ ☐
6. Correctly identified instrument #6 as a/an _____.	☐ ☐	☐ ☐
7. Correctly identified instrument #7 as a/an _____.	☐ ☐	☐ ☐
8. Correctly identified instrument #8 as a/an _____.	☐ ☐	☐ ☐
9. Correctly identified instrument #9 as a/an _____.	☐ ☐	☐ ☐
10. Correctly identified instrument #10 as a/an _____.	☐ ☐	☐ ☐

Student's score _____ _____

Evaluator's comments

Evaluation Form

Competency 30 - 2 *Preparing an Instrument Tray for an Extraction*

Performance Objective: Given an appropriate selection of surgical instruments, the student will select the instruments required for a single extraction. The student will state the use of each instrument. Sterile technique must be followed while preparing the tray.

Important: *The instructor will play the role of the dentist and identify the tooth to be extracted and specifying the instruments to be included on the tray. Appropriate PPE must also be available.*

Time limit: _____ Other conditions: _____

Points per step = _____ Maximum score = _____ Passing score = _____

*Check the left box **only** if step is performed correctly.*
Place score in the adjacent box.

	Evaluator #1		Evaluator #2	
1. Gathered appropriate supplies as specified on the instructor's instrumentation list.	☐	☐	☐	☐
2. Arranged the instruments in the sequence of use on the tray.	☐	☐	☐	☐
3. Maintained sterile technique while preparing the tray.	☐	☐	☐	☐
4. Stated the use of each instrument.	☐	☐	☐	☐
5. Covered the tray to protect it until used.	☐	☐	☐	☐
6. Followed the appropriate exposure control measures throughout the procedure.	☐	☐	☐	☐

Student's score   _____   _____

Evaluator's comments

Evaluation Form

Competency 31 - 1 *Creating Provisional Coverage*

Performance Objective: In states where it is legal, the student will create a temporary acrylic crown for a molar with a full crown preparation. This will be performed on a typodont or mannikin.

Time limit: _____ Other conditions: _____

Points per step = _____ Maximum score = _____ Passing score = _____

Check the left box **only** if step is performed correctly. Place score in the adjacent box.

	Evaluator #1		Evaluator #2	
1. Gathered appropriate supplies.	☐	☐	☐	☐
2. Obtained an acceptable alginate impression before the tooth was prepared.	☐	☐	☐	☐
3. Mixed the acrylic monomer and polymer.	☐	☐	☐	☐
4. Coated the prepared tooth with petroleum jelly or separating medium.	☐	☐	☐	☐
5. Placed the prepared acrylic dough into the impression in the area of the prepared tooth.	☐	☐	☐	☐
6. Placed the impression back in the "patient's" mouth.	☐	☐	☐	☐
7. Allowed the material to reach initial set.	☐	☐	☐	☐
8. Removed the tray from the patient's mouth and removed the temporary covering from the impression.	☐	☐	☐	☐
9. Trimmed excess material from the margins of the temporary covering.	☐	☐	☐	☐
10. Replaced the temporary covering on the prepared tooth and left it there until setting was complete.	☐	☐	☐	☐
11. Removed and evaluated the temporary coverage including the margins.	☐	☐	☐	☐
12. If the margins and/or the temporary were not acceptable, started over.	☐	☐	☐	☐
13. Smoothed the edges, made necessary adjustments, and completed the crown.	☐	☐	☐	☐
14. Followed the appropriate exposure control measures throughout the procedure.	☐	☐	☐	☐

Student's score _____ _____

Evaluator's comments

82

Evaluation Form

Competency 32 - 1 *Taking Alginate Impressions of Edentulous Arches*

Performance Objective: Working with edentulous models or stone diagnostic casts, the student will demonstrate taking an alginate impression of an edentulous mandibular arch and an edentulous maxillary arch.

Note: This procedure is to be performed only in those states where it is legal.

Time limit: _____ Other conditions: _____

Points per step = _____ Maximum score = _____ Passing score = _____

Check the left box **only** if step is performed correctly.
Place score in the adjacent box.

	Evaluator #1	Evaluator #2
1. Gathered appropriate supplies.	☐ ☐	☐ ☐
2. Explained the procedure to the patient.	☐ ☐	☐ ☐
Mandibular arch:		
3. Selected an appropriate tray.	☐ ☐	☐ ☐
4. Modified edges of tray with wax.	☐ ☐	☐ ☐
5. Mixed material and seated impression.	☐ ☐	☐ ☐
6. Described the use of fingers to gently massage the area of the face over the borders of the tray.	☐ ☐	☐ ☐
7. Removed and evaluated the completed impression.	☐ ☐	☐ ☐
Maxillary arch:		
8. Selected an appropriate tray.	☐ ☐	☐ ☐
9. Modified edges of tray with wax.	☐ ☐	☐ ☐
10. Mixed material and seated impression.	☐ ☐	☐ ☐
11. Described the use of fingers to gently massage the area of the face over the borders of the tray.	☐ ☐	☐ ☐
12. Removed and evaluated the completed impression.	☐ ☐	☐ ☐
13. Followed the appropriate exposure control measures throughout the procedure.	☐ ☐	☐ ☐

Student's score _____ _____

Evaluator's comments

Evaluation Form

Competency 33 - 1 *Making Telephone Calls in a Professional Manner*

Performance Objective: In a classroom simulation, the student will demonstrate calling a patient to confirm his dental appointment. Another student will play the patient.

Time limit: _____ *Other conditions:* _____

Points per step = _____ *Maximum score =* _____ *Passing score =* _____

*Check the left box **only** if step is performed correctly.*
Place score in the adjacent box.

	Evaluator #1		Evaluator #2	
1. Greeted the patient pleasantly. Determined that he or she had reached Ms. Chapman.	☐	☐	☐	☐
2. The assistant identified himself or herself appropriately.	☐	☐	☐	☐
3. The assistant briefly stated the reason for the call.	☐	☐	☐	☐
4. Took the appropriate steps when Ms. Chapman stated that she might not be able to keep the appointment.	☐	☐	☐	☐
5. If appropriate, scheduled a new appointment for Ms. Chapman.	☐	☐	☐	☐
6. Closed the conversation pleasantly and promptly.	☐	☐	☐	☐
7. Allowed Ms. Chapman to hang up first.	☐	☐	☐	☐
8. Managed the conversation in a professional manner.	☐	☐	☐	☐
9. Achieved the goal of either confirming or rescheduling the appointment.	☐	☐	☐	☐

Student's score _____ _____

Evaluator's comments

Evaluation Form

Competency 33 - 2 *Greeting an Arriving Patient*

Performance Objective: In a classroom simulation, the student will greet an arriving new patient, Maria Garcia, and ask her to complete a new patient registration and medical history form. Mrs. Garcia has brought her two small children with her. Other students play the roles of Mrs. Garcia and the children.

Time limit: _____ *Other conditions:* _____

Points per step = _____ *Maximum score =* _____ *Passing score =* _____

*Check the left box **only** if step is performed correctly.*
Place score in the adjacent box.

	Evaluator #1	Evaluator #2
1. Greeted the patient pleasantly and verified the patient's identity.	☐ ☐	☐ ☐
2. The assistant introduced him- or herself and welcomed Mrs. Garcia to the practice.	☐ ☐	☐ ☐
3. Explained the need for the information. Asked Mrs. Garcia to complete the required forms.	☐ ☐	☐ ☐
4. Suggested that there were toys available to amuse the children while Mrs. Garcia did this.	☐ ☐	☐ ☐
5. When Mrs. Garcia expressed difficulty completing the forms, offered to aid her in completing them.	☐ ☐	☐ ☐
6. Maintained a pleasant and professional attitude throughout the discussion.	☐ ☐	☐ ☐

Student's score _____ _____

Evaluator's comments

Evaluation Form

Competency 34 - 1 *Making Financial Arrangements*

Performance Objective: In a classroom simulation, the student will demonstrate making financial arrangements with a new patient. The patient is Mrs. DiNatale. Another student will play Mrs. DiNatale.

Time limit: _____ *Other conditions:* _____

Points per step = _____ *Maximum score =* _____ *Passing score =* _____

*Check the left box **only** if step is performed correctly.*
Place score in the adjacent box.

	Evaluator #1	Evaluator #2
1. Explained the need for treatment to Mrs. DiNatale.	☐ ☐	☐ ☐
2. Explained the available payment plans to Mrs. DiNatale.	☐ ☐	☐ ☐
3. Answered Mrs. DiNatale's questions politely and completely.	☐ ☐	☐ ☐
4. Arrived at an acceptable agreement with Mrs. DiNatale.	☐ ☐	☐ ☐
5. Asked Mrs. DiNatale to complete the necessary forms.	☐ ☐	☐ ☐
6. Maintained a pleasant and professional attitude throughout the discussion.	☐ ☐	☐ ☐

Student's score   _____   _____

Evaluator's comments

Evaluation Form

Competency 34 - 2 *Making a Collection Telephone Call*

Performance Objective: In a classroom simulation, the student will demonstrate making a telephone collection call. The call is to Mrs. Moses, who has fallen behind on her payments. Another student will play Mrs. Moses.

Time limit: _____ Other conditions: _____

Points per step = _____ Maximum score = _____ Passing score = _____

*Check the left box **only** if step is performed correctly.*
Place score in the adjacent box.

	Evaluator #1	Evaluator #2
1. Stated at what hour the phone call was being placed.	☐ ☐	☐ ☐
2. Determined that she was speaking to the responsible party (Mrs. Moses).	☐ ☐	☐ ☐
3. Identified herself, her employer, and the reason for the call.	☐ ☐	☐ ☐
4. Was polite, empathetic, and offered to help.	☐ ☐	☐ ☐
5. Worked out alternative payment arrangement with Mrs. Moses.	☐ ☐	☐ ☐
6. Maintained a professional attitude throughout the conversation.	☐ ☐	☐ ☐
7. Terminated the conversation pleasantly.	☐ ☐	☐ ☐
8. Recorded the arrangements for the alternative payment plan on the patient's financial record.	☐ ☐	☐ ☐

Student's score _____ _____

Evaluator's comments

Evaluation Form

Competency 36 - 1 *Being Interviewed for a Position as a Chairside Assistant*

Performance Objective: With the instructor or another student playing the role of the interviewer, the student will demonstrate interviewing for a position as a chairside assistant.

Important: Before the interview, the student will have prepared and submitted to the interviewer a letter of application and a résumé.

Time limit: _____	Other conditions: _____
Points per step = _____	Maximum score = _____ Passing score = _____

*Check the left box **only** if step is performed correctly.*
Place score in the adjacent box.

	Evaluator #1	Evaluator #2
1. The applicant was dressed appropriately for an interview. As an alternative, she may describe appropriate dress.	☐ ☐	☐ ☐
2. The applicant's letter of application was neat and contained the appropriate information.	☐ ☐	☐ ☐
3. The applicant's résumé was well organized and professional in appearance.	☐ ☐	☐ ☐
4. The applicant answered the interviewer's questions.	☐ ☐	☐ ☐
5. The applicant asked appropriate questions.	☐ ☐	☐ ☐
6. The applicant made a good, professional impression.	☐ ☐	☐ ☐
7. At the end of the interview, the applicant thanked the interviewer.	☐ ☐	☐ ☐

Student's score _____ _____

Evaluator's comments